Diseases of Domestic Guinea Pigs

Second Edition

T0203088

LIBRARY OF VETERINARY PRACTICE

SERIES EDITORS
J.B. SUTTON, JP, MRCVS
S.T. SWIFT, MA, Vet MB, CertSAC, MRCVS

Also by V.C.G. Richardson:

Rabbits
Health, Husbandry and Diseases
ISBN 10: 0-632-05221-X
ISBN 13: 978-0632-05221-9

Diseases of Small Domestic Rodents
Second Edition
ISBN 10: 1-4051-0921-1
ISBN 13: 978-14051-0921-5

LIBRARY OF VETERINARY PRACTICE

Diseases of Domestic Guinea Pigs

Second Edition

V.C.G. Richardson

MA VetMB MRCVS

Blackwell
Science

Editorial offices:
Blackwell Science Ltd, 9600 Garsington Road, Oxford OX4 2DQ, UK
Tel: +44 (0) 1865 776868
Blackwell Publishing Inc., 350 Main Street, Malden, MA 02148-5020, USA
Tel: +1 781 388 8250
Blackwell Science Asia Pty Ltd, 550 Swanston Street, Carlton, Victoria 3053, Australia
Tel: +61 (0)3 8359 1011

First published 1992
Reprinted 1996 (twice), 1998
Second edition published 2000
Reprinted 2003, 2004, 2005

Library of Congress Cataloging-in-Publication Data is available

ISBN-10: 0-632-05209-0
ISBN-13: 978-0632-05209-7

A catalogue record for this title is available from the British Library

Set in 10/13.5pt Souvenir
by DP Photosetting, Aylesbury, Bucks

The publisher's policy is to use permanent paper from mills that operate a sustainable forestry policy, and which has been manufactured from pulp processed using acid-free and elementary chlorine-free practices. Furthermore, the publisher ensures that the text paper and cover board used have met acceptable environmental accreditation standards.

For further information on Blackwell Publishing, visit our website:
www.blackwellpublishing.com

CONTENTS

PREFACE

I have bred and exhibited guinea pigs for over 30 years, and since I qualified as a veterinary surgeon I have been able to expand this interest in a more professional capacity. This book aims to provide a comprehensive text covering all aspects of the species, and it is written in part to try and help dispel the myth that 'a sick guinea pig is a dead guinea pig'. It is hoped that it will be of help to veterinary surgeons in general practice, and also to anyone who shares an interest in guinea pigs.

The scientific name of the guinea pig is *Cavia porcellus*, from which their other name, the cavy, originates. When I was reviewing the references in preparation for this book 'guinea pig' emerged as the most popular term and that is why I have chosen to use it throughout my text.

I have tried to make the information as readily accessible as possible, and wherever a treatment is mentioned it is given a reference number in brackets. All these treatments are listed numerically in Chapter 11 which provides full details of dose rates, contraindications, etc., and also the components of the proprietary preparations which should enable like alternatives to be found, if the former are unavailable.

There are many people whom I would like to thank: those who have given me advice on some of the treatments mentioned, my many friends and fellow exhibitors, and especially my colleague and husband Ean, for his patience, encouragement and help in preparing the manuscript. I am also grateful to Wayne Chant for providing the illustrations.

V.C.G.R.

1 THE SKIN

The skin of the guinea pig normally provides a resistant barrier against infection. However, there are many factors which lower this resistance and predispose the guinea pig to the development of skin disease. One of the most common findings is an increased incidence of skin problems in guinea pigs fed on marginal diets, especially if these diets have a low vitamin C content. The feeding of stale dried food will cause such a problem as the vitamin C content deteriorates rapidly 6–9 weeks after milling. Rabbit food is also too low in vitamin C to be used as a staple diet for guinea pigs. If guinea pigs are fed a rabbit food their diet must be supplemented with daily greenfood and carrots, and if necessary with vitamin C in their drinking water.

Other important stresses which predispose the guinea pig to the development of skin conditions are overheating, pregnancy and showing.

SPECIFIC SKIN CONDITIONS

Ringworm

Clinical signs: Areas of alopecia, usually accompanied by varying degrees of seborrhoea. The lesions are often found around the face but may spread to the rest of the body. The affected hair can be readily plucked from its follicles. The condition may or may not be pruritic. There may also be accompanying lesions on the owner.

Diagnosis: The causal agent is usually *Tricophyton mentagrophytes* or *Microsporum gypseum* so it will not fluoresce under ultraviolet light (Wood's lamp). Direct microscopic examination of hair from the lesion together with culture on Sabouraud's medium will confirm the diagnosis.

Treatment: Griseofulvin (Tx 18) at a dose of 25 mg/kg (approximately 0.75 mg/kg of feed) for 4–6 weeks is generally effective. If griseofulvin is used to treat an individual animal it is best given orally on a daily basis, and the approximate dose is one-eighth of a tablet daily, which can be given mixed with an unsaturated fatty acid supplement (e.g. 0.5 ml Norderm, Norden Laboratories). Care must be taken when using griseofulvin in very young animals (under 3 months) as a high incidence of infant mortality has been reported in association with the use of this anti-fungal preparation in one colony. Griseofulvin should also not be administered to pregnant sows.

Alternatively tolnaftate 1% (Tx 19, Tinaderm-M cream) can be applied to the lesions twice daily until they resolve.

Cases with severe accompanying seborrhoea will benefit from the use of an anti-fungal shampoo, e.g. hexetidine 0.5% (Tx 40). This shampoo is most effective if it is left in contact with the skin for some time (1–2 hours in severely affected cases) before rinsing. Alternatively the guinea pig can be dipped in a 0.2% solution of enilconazole (Tx 17).

A diet with good vitamin C content must be fed at the same time as treating with any anti-fungal agent to enable the affected guinea pig to make a full recovery.

Other mycoses

Clinical signs: Guinea pigs may suffer from a range of other mycotic infections, and the clinical signs may vary from mild skin changes indistinguishable from mange in its early stages, to very severe seborrhoea with accompanying systemic signs including cystitis, pneumonia, convulsions and reproductive disorders.

Diagnosis: Microscopic examination of the hair and culture on Sabouraud's medium.

Cases which are suggestive of mycotic infection are those which do not respond to the standard anti-parasitic treatment.

Treatment: Griseofulvin (as for ringworm) and the use of an anti-fungal shampoo, e.g. 0.5% hexetidine (Tx 40). The shampoo should be left in contact with the skin for as long as possible (up to 2 hours) before rinsing. The effectiveness of the treatment will be increased if all the affected hairs are plucked from the guinea pig's body as this will remove a high percentage of the fungal spores. This treatment can be repeated every 3–4 days as necessary.

The use of amphotericin B has been reported in those cases exhibiting severe systemic involvement.

Mange

This condition may also be called 'sellnick' or 'rat mange'. It refers to the condition produced by *Trixacarus caviae*, a sarcoptiform mite.

Clinical signs: These usually occur 3–5 weeks after infection, although they may remain inapparent for considerable periods. The lesions are seen mainly around the head and shoulders and over the dorsum, but may spread further to affect the whole guinea pig. The hair comes out and the skin is seborrhoeic and usually intensely pruritic. There may also be many open sores due to self-trauma. If the sow is in-pig and is quite severely affected she may resorb or abort her litter. If her young are born normally they will become infected immediately.

In cases where the pruritus is severe the guinea pig may also exhibit nervous signs, and in extreme cases may actually have fits.

Diagnosis: Microscopic examination of skin scrapings.

Treatment: Numerous treatments have been advocated. Probably the most effective is ivermectin (Tx 31), but as this is not licensed for guinea pigs it should be used with care. The dose is 200 µg/kg and this can be repeated at 10–14-day intervals if necessary. The Ivomec injection (Merial Animal Health Ltd.) is the most convenient preparation to use (0.02 ml/kg) and it can be diluted 1 : 10 to produce a dose of 0.2 ml which should be administered subcutaneously. Alternatively this same drug has been administered orally with the same effect. Up to 2 drops from a 2 ml syringe (equivalent to 400 µg) can be given with no side-effects. Although the oral absorption of ivermectin has not been evaluated, treatment in this way seems to be effective.

Trials using ivermectin, performed at the Cambridge Cavy Trust have shown that greater doses of this drug can be used without any adverse effects. Their recommendations are as follows:

- Age 3 weeks to 3 months: 0.1 ml (1000 µg) by subcutaneous injection. Oral dosing is not recommended.
- Age 3 months to adult: 0.2 ml by subcutaneous injection. One drop given orally.

These treatments can be repeated after an interval of 10–14 days.

Other preparations which can be used include sprays containing pyre-thrum extract (e.g. Johnson's Anti-Pest Insect spray). Seleen (Tx 30) can be used as a shampoo.

If this or any other skin condition is accompanied by intense pruritus, this can be controlled by an injection of a steroid preparation (Tx 37 and 38). Creams containing local anaesthetic agents can also be used on the lesions to prevent self-trauma.

Self-trauma can also be limited if the hind feet are lightly dressed, or alternatively the worst sores can be protected with a loose body bandage.

If nervous signs are present, diazepam (Tx 44) at a dose of 1–2 mg/kg can be given intramuscularly to help control these. However, if the symptoms are as severe as this, euthanasia may have to be considered.

An alternative treatment for controlling any seizures is primidone (Mysoline Tx 42).

If a pregnant sow is badly affected she should be treated. The slight risks incurred by handling a gravid sow are better than the consequences of leaving her untreated. Ivermectin has been administered during pregnancy without obvious side effects, and dosing is a less stressful procedure than bathing or dipping.

If the problem is a recurrent one, treatment is more effective if it is varied. If the same preparation is used repeatedly it is not unknown for some mites to develop resistance to the treatment and the condition then becomes more persistent.

The environment should also be treated. The hutch can be sprayed with an environmental flea spray.

Comment: Trixacarus caviae is a burrowing mite, and transmission can be via direct or indirect contact. The female burrows into the skin and lays her eggs in the tunnels she creates. Multiple larvae then hatch out in these tunnels, metamorphose through two nymph stages and then develop into adults. The life cycle takes 14 days. The mite eggs can remain dormant for a period of 1–21 months, and can exist all this time in the host. Stresses such as malnutrition, overcrowding, poor ventilation, extreme heat and pregnancy predispose to this condition.

Prevention: If there is a problem in the caviary all individuals can be treated with ivermectin (Tx 31) given orally in order to eradicate any sub-clinical disease.

Demodex

Clinical signs: Areas of alopecia, especially around the head and forelegs. The condition may or may not be pruritic.

Diagnosis: Microscopic examination of skin scrapings.

Treatment: Injection of a high dose of ivermectin (Tx 31) which may need to be repeated two or three times at fortnightly intervals.

Lice

Clinical signs: This condition need not be pruritic, and the lice can often be seen in the fur. 'Static lice' refers to the eggs of the lice which are seen as black or white specks sticking to the hair, especially around the neck and ears and on the ventral abdomen. 'Running lice' refers to the adult forms which are visible to the naked eye.

In some cases the term static lice is used to describe the fur mite *Chirodiscoides caviae* (see below).

Diagnosis: Microscopic examination of hair and skin scrapings.

Treatment: A spray containing pyrethrum extract (e.g. Johnson's Anti-Pest Insect spray). Seleen (Tx 30) will also be effective, and treatment can be repeated at weekly intervals. A more old-fashioned remedy was to use oil of sassafras, but unfortunately this oil is no longer readily obtainable. It can be worked gently into the coat avoiding the eyes and genitals, and left to evaporate. It will kill the lice and their eggs and leave the coat in a glossy condition. The treatment can be repeated after 14 days. Alternatively, a human head lice preparation containing malathion can be used. The spirit based preparation can be rubbed into the coat, and left for at least 10 minutes before combing with a fine comb. The guinea pig should be rinsed in warm water and dried.

Comment: Causal agents are varied. Infestations with *Gyropus ovalis, Trimenopen jenningsi* and *Gliricola porcelli* have been recorded.

Gliricola porcelli is the most common. The adults are yellow-grey in colour and are up to 1.5 mm long. *Gyropus ovalis* are similar, but are slightly smaller and they have a less rounded head. *Trimenopen jenningsi* is thought to be of little pathogenic significance unless the guinea pig is stressed.

Fur mite

These mites (*Chirodiscoides caviae*) are 0.5 mm long and are often found joined in pairs. They appear to produce no clinical signs even when the guinea pig is heavily infested. They will be removed with any of the ectoparasitic treatments recommended above for mange and lice.

Prevention: The load of ectoparasites can be reduced by hanging a Vapona sticky strip (containing dichlorvos) in the environment for a 48-hour period once a week. Nuvan Top, a spray containing dichlorvos for use in cats and dogs, *should not* be used on guinea pigs. The active ingredients are powerful cholinesterase inhibitors and toxicity is likely to develop. If Nuvan Top has been used the antidote is atropine sulphate which should be administered at a dose of 0.1 mg/kg given intraperitoneally.

Rabbit fur mite

The rabbit fur mite *Psoroptes cuniculi* has been isolated from skin lesions in a guinea pig. The ears, face, underbody and hind legs were affected by a crusting and scaling dermatitis which was extremely pruritic. Treatment with three doses of ivermectin at 10 day intervals was effective.

'Broken back'

Clinical sign: A single area of hair loss in the centre of the back which may become an open sore; if left will scab over. This condition is often mistakenly assumed to be mange. It seems to be associated with stresses such as showing or pregnancy.

Treatment: Bathe the sore with a dilute saline solution (Tx 52) and dry. Dermisol cream or Vetsovate (Tx 23 or 26) can be applied topically up to three times daily. However, the condition will resolve with bathing only. Once the lesion is healed the affected skin may be fairly dry and this can be conditioned by topical application of cod-liver oil or evening primrose oil.

Comment: This condition affects lighter coloured guinea pigs most frequently, and it is thought to occur as a result of the guinea pig 'overheating'. Barley is a particularly 'overheating food' as is flaked maize, and these should be removed from the diet. An excess of rabbit pellets has also been implicated as a cause of overheating. The problem is seen at its worst in the heat of the summer.

'Post-natal sores'

This condition is similar to 'broken back' and develops in some sows after parturition as a sore in the centre of the back, and it can be treated in the same manner. It is thought to be due to a mineral and protein deficiency.

In late pregnancy sows prone to developing this condition can be given some Bemax as a supplement sprinkled on their food. Alternatively they can be given a bread and milk mash to which extra soya flour has been added to provide supplementary protein. A couple of drops of Vitapet daily as a source of polyunsaturated fatty acids may also be beneficial. This condition will also respond if 1–2 drops of Abidec (Tx 45), a vitamin preparation, are given orally once a day.

Comment: This condition also occurs in sows during gestation and is also likely to be due to a mineral and protein deficiency. The treatment is the same as for 'broken back'.

Skin lesions immediately after parturition

Clinical signs: Sows develop raw patches on their rumps and ventral abdomen soon after parturition.

Comment: This condition is more prevalent if the sow has had a long and difficult labour. She becomes caked in blood and uterine fluids because she is too tired to clean herself immediately after the birth. This then begins to irritate her and she tears the hair out from the affected area; the lesions are therefore due to self-trauma.

There is also a possible inherited tendency towards developing this condition.

Treatment: It is important to check the sow after the birth and if necessary clean her with a dilute solution of Savlon (Tx 51).

If raw patches do develop they must be cleaned gently and towelled dry. Antibiotic creams should be used with extreme caution as there is a real risk that they will be ingested by the youngsters whilst suckling and therefore these preparations are probably best avoided. If the sores are weeping, calamine lotion can be applied and this should dry up the lesions in 24 hours with less risk to the youngsters. Some sources suggest the application of cod-liver oil to the bald areas to help them heal, but this should be avoided due to the risk of vitamin D overdose if ingested by the suckling youngsters.

Seborrhoea

Seborrhoea and the presence of excess scurf in the coat may be a symptom of many different conditions, notably mange, ringworm and other mycotic infections, and chronic liver disorders. The presence of this scurf is in itself intensely pruritic irrespective of the causal agent.

Treatment: As well as treating the underlying cause, the scurf can be removed by using a tar-based shampoo, e.g. Tarlite (Tx 43). Shampooing can be repeated at weekly intervals and the resultant improvement will bring great relief to the affected guinea pig.

If it is difficult to determine whether the initiating cause is parasitic or fungal in origin it is advisable to use Seleen (Tx 30) which has both anti-parasitic and antifungal properties.

Alopecia

During pregnancy

Some sows lose their hair during pregnancy. The symptoms begin in middle to late pregnancy and the hair just begins to fall out. There is no accompanying pruritus. If a sow has experienced this condition once she is likely to do so during subsequent pregnancies, and the condition is also worse in older and frequently bred females.

Treatment: Vitamin B supplementation has been advocated, either in the form of a weekly multivitamin injection or as daily drops of an oral preparation. However, the condition will resolve slowly after parturition without treatment.

Hormonal

A bilateral symmetrical alopecia may be seen in older sows associated with ovarian cysts. These cysts may reach 2–3 cm in diameter and are readily identified during abdominal palpation.

Treatment: Ovariohysterectomy. Alternatively, the cysts can be drained via percutaneous needle aspiration.

Post-natal

After parturition some sows may lose most of their coat. The hair is lost bilaterally from the flanks and ventral abdomen.

Occasionally the young may actually be responsible for pulling hair from their dams.

Treatment: None is required. This condition is thought to be hormonal in origin and will correct itself once the sow stops nursing her litter.

Liver disease

Clinical signs: The hair cover is sparse and the skin may be thickened. There is often accompanying seborrhoea. Pruritus is not usually a feature unless the seborrhoea is severe. The guinea pig may twitch frequently.

Severe, untreated mycosis will also present with similar clinical signs.

Treatment: If parasitic and fungal causes are eliminated then this condition is often a sign of underlying liver disease. If the seborrhoea is intense, a tar and sulphur based shampoo (Tarlite Tx 43) is very effective and this can be repeated weekly as necessary. Other treatment is supportive, and should include a vitamin and polyunsaturated fatty acid supplement, e.g. Vitapet. However, in severe cases exhibiting nervous signs the prognosis is poor.

Scurvy

One of the manifestations of this condition is hair loss, usually accompanied by the other symptoms of weight loss, lameness, weakness and bleeding from the gums.

Treatment: Vitamin C at a dose of 100 mg/kg, preferably given orally in drop form, until the condition resolves.

Comment: In any skin condition the provision of adequate vitamin C is of paramount importance. Plenty of this vitamin is to be found in fresh greens, carrots and beetroot. Rosehip syrup is another useful source of vitamin C. (For further details about this vitamin refer to Chapter 9.)

Hair loss at weaning

Young guinea pigs may get a thin hair coat at weaning time as they lose their neonatal haircoat and it is gradually replaced by mature hair. No treatment is required other than the provision of an adequate diet, as this is a completely natural phenomenon.

Chewing

Clinical signs: Hair loss in any area of the body, and the hair is often bitten to the roots. It may be self-inflicted in which case only the areas the guinea pig can reach are affected, or it may be more widespread if the chewing is from other guinea pigs. Guinea pigs that share accommodation with rabbits are often chewed by the rabbit. In one case of a guinea pig kept in an outside run the hair was seen being removed by a robin to provide nesting material!

Treatment: If the condition is self-inflicted it is often a result of boredom, and alteration of the guinea pig's environment may break the habit. As, by its nature, the guinea pig is always eating, the provision of ample amounts of good hay will help prevent boredom and stop the development of this vice. If the chewing is being done by other guinea pigs, the affected individual should be penned separately. If the hair loss is found in youngsters as a result of overgrooming by their mother, the affected young should be weaned as soon as possible.

In some cases of coat chewing in the long-haired breeds (Peruvians, Coronets and Shelties) a vitamin and mineral deficiency has been implicated and these cases have been resolved once 'Stress', a supplement for dogs and cats, has been added to the daily diet.

Urine scalding

Clinical signs: A moist dermatitis around the genitals ventrally in the female and around the rump in the male. It may be a consequence of polyuria.

Treatment: Twice-daily applications of a combined antibiotic–steroid preparation such as Vetsovate cream (Tx 26) is effective. The affected area can be protected by use of a resistant barrier cream such as zinc and castor oil, or Vaseline.

Epidermoid cyst (sebaceous cyst)

Clinical signs: These cysts can arise anywhere on the body, but are usually found on the back. They are slightly soft when squeezed, and if ruptured they discharge their caseous contents.

Treatment: If the cyst ruptures it can be squeezed out and then bathed with a mild saline solution (Tx 52). No extra treatment is needed. If the cysts are irritating the guinea pig then their removal should be considered, although they may recur subsequently. Otherwise they can be left.

Comment: These cysts are derived from hair follicles (not sebaceous glands) and possess a keratinizing epidermal lining which generates the caseous contents.

Abscesses

These may occur anywhere on the body and are often the result of fighting. They must be differentiated from cervical lymphadenitis (see Chapter 7) and pseudotuberculosis. Occasionally a pea-sized lump is felt in the throat which is due to a swollen lymph node, and this will regress with time.

A wide range of bacteria have been isolated from such abscesses including *Pseudomonas aeruginosa*, *Pasteurella multocida*, *Corynebacterium pyogenes*, *Staphylococcus aureus*, *Streptococcus* spp. and other environmental contaminants (*Enterobacteriaceae*).

Clinical signs: A localized soft swelling originating from a cut or scratch. It may be hot and painful to the touch. Abscesses commonly occur in the throat region where they are usually the result of a thistle from the hay penetrating through the mucous membranes of the mouth and tracking under the chin.

Treatment: If the abscess has burst it must be thoroughly bathed with a dilute saline solution (Tx 52), and flushed with a 3% solution of hydrogen peroxide (Tx 49). It is then best to use anti-bacterials topically only, either a cream e.g. Dermisol (Tx 23), or perhaps more conveniently an intra-mammary preparation to instil antibiotics into the abscess site. The latter has the advantage of a long nozzle to get the antibiotics under the skin, even when the wound has closed to a hole of small diameter. If care is taken to use only a small amount of an intramammary preparation (considering its high antibiotic concentration) the response to treatment will be good.

If the abscess has not burst, it can be brought to a head with warm poulticing, by smearing warm magnesium sulphate paste onto the surface of the abscess, or by lancing with a scalpel blade.

The affected guinea pig must be isolated to prevent other guinea pigs licking the abscess and ingesting the infected material.

Comment: Two adult boars should never be penned together as they will usually fight. However, an older boar may tolerate a younger one if there are no females around, and two sibling males may tolerate each other if kept together from birth, but again only if they are alone. It is therefore better to keep a pair of females, as females will nearly always live together in harmony.

As abscesses may also arise from scratches caused by sharp flooring or wire doors, or even sharp foodstuffs, e.g. straw, it is important to eliminate these from the hutch to prevent the problem from recurring.

Boils

Clinical signs: These may occur anywhere on the body and appear as subcutaneous fluid-filled swellings. Agoutis seem to be particularly prone to developing this condition.

Treatment: None is necessary: the fluid may resorb or burst on its own. The temptation to drain boils should be resisted as there is a likelihood of introducing infection.

Grease gland (scent gland)

This is a wrinkled piece of skin at the base of the spine which is not normally noticeable as it is covered with hair. It sometimes becomes very thick and glutinous due to the grease it secretes. It is much more noticeable in boars than sows, and it can become quite dirty. However, it is perfectly normal and is best left alone.

If necessary the thick grease can be removed with surgical spirit or a gel hand cleanser (e.g. Swarfega).

Anal fold dermatitis

Clinical signs: A moist dermatitis in the circumanal skin folds, caused by a build up of secretions of sebum in these folds and subsequent secondary infection.

Treatment: The area should be cleaned with an anti-bacterial agent and then a topical anti-bacterial cream, e.g. Panolog (Tx 25) or Dermisol (Tx 23) can be applied two or three times daily until the condition resolves.

Basal cell tumour

Clinical signs: A slow growing mass, which is roughly oval, well-circumscribed, firmly attached to the epidermis, but freely mobile over the underlying tissues. As the mass increases in size it may ulcerate through the skin discharging some of its caeseous contents, and at this time it may become secondarily infected. They can be found anywhere on the body, but are usually seen in the skin of the dorsum or flanks.

Treatment: Surgical excision of the mass will result in a complete cure. If the tumour is entirely resected local recurrence and metastases are rare.

Pathology: Basal cell tumours contain variable degrees of differentiation, and they can differentiate into both squamous epithelium and sebaceous cells. Some cells in the centre may form hair follicle-like structures with a clearly defined zone of mature keratin, and these tumours are termed tri-cofolliculomas.

Comment: These skin tumours are seen fairly frequently, and there may be a familial tendency to their development. They are benign tumours, but it is advisable to remove them before they ulcerate.

Fly strike (blowfly myiasis)

Clinical signs: The presence of larvae (maggots) of blowfly colonizing a moist wound. Maggots may also be found under the adjacent skin.

Treatment: Thorough cleansing of the area (Tx 49, 50) and removal of all the maggots. Subsequently the wound must be kept clean and dry, and an anti-bacterial cream can be applied (Tx 23).

Comment: This condition is relatively uncommon in guinea pigs. However, if the wound is cleaned aggressively and all the maggots removed, the prognosis for recovery is good. Guinea pigs, unlike rabbits, seem far less susceptible to the development of the toxic shock associated with the larval secretions.

2 THE REPRODUCTIVE SYSTEM

ANATOMY

Figures 2.1 and 2.2 describe the internal anatomy of the reproductive tract of both sexes. An important consideration is that in males the inguinal canals which contain the testes are open throughout the guinea pig's life, and therefore there is an increased tendency for prolapse of the abdominal organs after castration. In the adult male, the coiled tubular vesicular glands lie ventral to the urethra and extend to a length of approximately 10 cm into the abdominal cavity from their base in the pubic area. They should not be confused with the uterine horns of the female.

There are two mammary glands and the nipples, situated in the groin, are present in both sexes. For details of the external genitalia see Fig. 2.3.

Sexing

This can be done at any age. The guinea pig is turned onto its back and its weight should be supported with the palm of one hand so that the genitalia can be examined. In both sexes the anus is closely associated to the genitalia. Gentle pressure on either side of the male's sex organs will extrude the penis, whereas in front of the anus in the sow there is a hairless area of skin shaped like an upside-down 'Y' covering the vagina. In front of the vagina is the urethral opening. The vagina is normally closed by a membrane (the hymen) except during oestrus and at parturition.

When the male's penis is extruded there should be two prongs of even length at the end. If these are absent or of unequal length the boar is likely to be sterile.

14

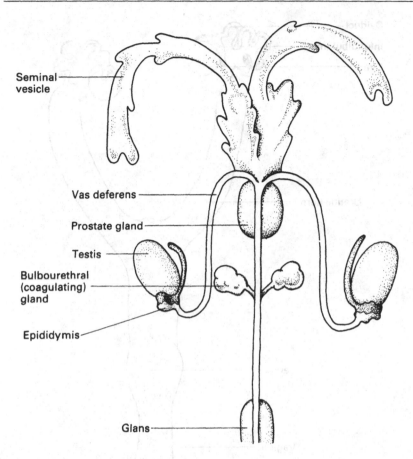

Fig. 2.1   The male reproductive tract.

Seminal vesicle

Vas deferens

Prostate gland

Testis

Bulbourethral (coagulating) gland

Epididymis

Glans

REPRODUCTIVE PHYSIOLOGY

Reproductive parameters of the guinea pig

- Sexual maturity (female): 4–6 weeks
- Sexual maturity (male): 3–5 weeks
- Female breeding age: 4–5 months, weight 500 g
- Male breeding age: 3–5 months, weight 550 g
- Oestrus cycle: 15–17 days
- Gestation range: 59–72 days (depending upon litter size)
- Litter size: 1–6 (average 3)
- Birthweight: 100 g each
- Breeding life of female: 4–5 years

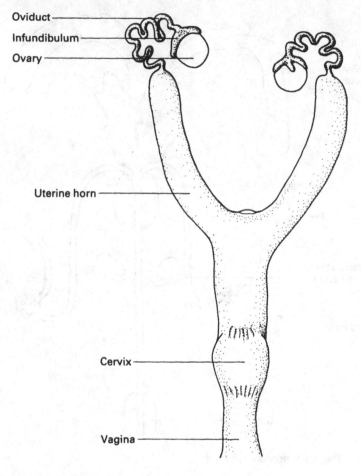

Fig. 2.2   The female reproductive tract.

- Breeding life of male: 5 years or longer
- Weaning age: 3 weeks

Breeding

A female can be put with a male once she weighs 500 g, or is 4–5 months old. However, she should have her first litter before she reaches 10 months of age, because soon after this time her pelvic bones fuse and her chances of developing dystocia are greatly increased.

Although males are capable of breeding from 4 weeks of age, it is advisable not to use them for breeding until they are over 4 months old. Guinea pigs can either be kept as breeding pairs or as a harem. One male

Fig. 2.3 External genitalia.

can be run with four or five females at the same time, but two males should never be put together in a large pen of females.

If males are not allowed to mate with a female until they are a year old, their libido will decrease, even to the extent that they may become infertile, and for this reason it is advisable that they are bred from as soon as they are over 4 months of age.

Oestrus

Guinea pigs are polyoestrus, coming into season every 15–17 days, and at this time they exhibit several characteristic changes in their behaviour patterns. The sow may mount other females in the pen and give a purring or mating call as she does this. If she is stroked along the back and rump at this time she will dip her back and purr (the lordosis posture).

Oestrus itself lasts for 24–48 hours, and the sow will accept the boar for approximately 6–11 hours during this time. Spontaneous ovulation usually occurs 10 hours after the onset of oestrus. As the sow comes into season her external genitalia swell, and the hymen usually opens the day before oestrus to allow for copulation with the boar. Once the mating has been completed the vagina is sealed by a plug of ejaculate known as the stopper, and this generally remains in place for 48 hours after which time it drops out and the hymen reseals until parturition.

Post-partum oestrus

Sows return to oestrus 6–48 hours after parturition, so it is wise to separate the sow and the boar once the sow is pregnant to avoid her being mated again at this time. Carrying a second litter whilst rearing the first would be harmful. (At this time 80% of matings are fertile.)

PREGNANCY

Gestation ranges from 59 to 72 days depending upon the size of the litter. If the litter is large the gestation is likely to be shorter, whereas conversely smaller litters are carried for a longer time.

The size of the litter is determined by the sow, and there is an inherited tendency to produce either large or small litters. The optimum litter size is three. Very small litters (one or two young) carry an increased chance of dystocia due to foetal oversize, whereas large litters lead to the birth of small and often weakly youngsters.

Pregnancy diagnosis

Pregnancy can be determined by monitoring the sow's weight, as there is usually a considerable increase during gestation, often up to twice her normal weight. However handling, and therefore weighing, of the pregnant sow must be kept to the minimum to avoid any possible complications during her pregnancy. By careful abdominal palpation the first foetal movements can be felt at 42 days (these first movements are termed 'quickening') and at 50 days very definite movements can be felt. These continue throughout gestation until the last week when the uterus has become so gravid that the movement of the foetuses becomes restricted and in some cases may not be felt at all.

This examination must be undertaken very gently, the sow being held around the shoulders with one hand whilst her abdomen rests on the palm of the other hand. No digital pressure is necessary, the movements will be felt if the palm is cupped around the sow's body.

From 6 weeks of gestation foetal skeletons are visible radiographically, but radiography should not be necessary to detect pregnancy and may be harmful if inadvertently done before this date. However, radiography or ultrasound can be useful to check sows that are overdue (those that have been over 70 days without a boar), as in some cases a sow may resorb all or part of a litter but still continue to look pregnant.

Superfetation

This phenomenon has been recorded in guinea pigs. It is possible for the sow to carry foetuses from two separate fertilization events occurring at different oestruses. In most cases a second fertile mating occurs at the subsequent oestrus; however, in several cases sows have produced two litters 35 days apart (the second litter being produced from fertilized ova shed two oestrus cycles later). The uterus has two separate horns and each litter is carried in a different horn. It is quite possible for both litters to be reared successfully.

Pseudopregnancy

This condition is rare but has been recorded in guinea pigs. Its duration is approximately 17 days.

Sows which miscarry their litters early in gestation may continue to look pregnant and may actually begin to produce milk. Despite the absence of young such sows may produce milk for 1–2 weeks, and great care must be taken to ensure that they do not develop mastitis during this time. If the sow is not fed any greens her milk flow will soon decrease, and it is advisable to withhold all such green food until the condition resolves.

Special nutritional considerations of the pregnant sow

(1) During her pregnancy the sow's requirements for vitamin C increases twofold from 10 mg/kg/day to 20 mg/kg/day. This can be supplied by adding soluble vitamin C tablets (e.g. Redoxon Tx 47) to the drinking water (the average guinea pig drinks 85 ml/day). Alternatively, rosehip syrup or blackcurrant juice can be added to the water bottles. However, most commercial pellets will provide adequate vitamin C provided that they have not been stored for a prolonged period (greater than 3 months). Beetroot and carrots contain 3 mg per 25 g of vitamin C, and most cabbages, broccoli and spinach 17 mg per 25 g of vitamin C, so supplementation may only be necessary in the winter when green food is scarce. Youngsters born to vitamin C deficient mothers may have paralysed hindquarters and swollen painful joints.

(2) It is important that the sow does not become obese as this will predispose her to developing pregnancy toxaemia. She must be allowed access to plenty of good hay and grass which will be filling but of less

calorific value than concentrates. Eating large quantities of molasses-enriched food will similarly lead to obesity, as will flaked maize which is very calorific. She must not be kept in cramped surroundings but encouraged to exercise.

(3) Raspberry leaves are often fed by breeders during gestation and are said to ensure ease of parturition. Various raspberry products are certainly used for this reason in other species and the author feels that they are a useful supplement during pregnancy. They also have mild astringent properties.

(4) Bran fed in the form of a mash is a useful component of the diet, but care must be taken not to overfeed this cereal as it is high in phosphorus and low in calcium and will lead to the development of weak young with undermineralized skeletons.

Complications during pregnancy

Pregnancy toxaemia

Clinical signs: The sow stops eating, becomes depressed, and adopts a hunched, ruffled appearance. She may salivate profusely and the characteristic smell of ketones can be detected on her breath as she becomes ketoacidotic. The condition progresses to muscle spasms and death. The symptoms often occur abruptly, and the condition is more prevalent in hot weather.

Pathology: Laboratory findings include aciduria, proteinuria and hyperlipaemia. Microscopically there is a fatty degeneration of the liver and at post-mortem this organ looks pale yellow and is enlarged and very friable. The blood is lactescent (fatty) and the adrenal glands may be enlarged and haemorrhagic.

Treatment: Treatment is rarely successful in advanced cases. In the early stages administration of a glucose or propylene glycol solution may prove beneficial (e.g. Ketol). In later stages an injection of steroids such as betamethasone or dexamethasone (Tx 37 and 38) and administration of up to 10 ml fluids subcutaneously (4% or 5% glucose – saline Tx 15) can be attempted. An intramuscular injection of vitamin B_{12} (Tx 48) may act as an effective appetite stimulant.

Comment: Pregnancy toxaemia is a metabolic disorder similar to that observed in sheep before parturition (twin lamb disease). Predisposing factors are obesity and any stress which may induce temporary anorexia in late pregnancy. The sow goes into negative energy balance. She is unable to supply sufficient glucose to the developing foetuses from the products of digestion and begins to catabolize her own tissues. This progresses to the development of ketoacidosis. It is therefore very important to keep stresses such as handling and weighing to the absolute mininum.

There is evidence to suggest that sub-clinical hypocalcaemia may predispose to the development of ketosis, and calcium supplementation during the last week of pregnancy and first week of lactation will reduce the incidence of this disease.

Ketosis and an associated hepatic lipidosis is also seen in obese animals and older males after stress. The treatment is the same as for the pregnant sow.

Prevention: The sow must be housed in a hutch large enough to provide room for exercise and must not be allowed to become obese. The nest area, the food and water should be kept as far apart as possible so that the sow has to keep moving. In-pig sows can be given water in which a little glucose has been dissolved as a ready supply of this sugar in late pregnancy. An alternative preventative measure is to add a small amount of liquid Lectade to the drinking water of pregnant sows (this product is also used to treat twin lamb disease in sheep). The required dilution of this is 20 ml of Lectade into 250 ml of water (Tx 16).

Calcium supplementation (Tx 46) can be given orally during the last week of pregnancy and the first week of lactation.

Resorption

Clinical signs: This may occur before pregnancy has been detected and therefore go unnoticed, it just being assumed that the sow is taking her time in conceiving, or that she is infertile. Any stress such as a sudden diet change may lead to resorption, as will a period of poor feeding. Sows with severe mange mite infestation are quite likely either to resorb or abort their litters. If foetal loss occurs in the very early stages of gestation the sow may not outwardly appear sick.

Treatment: Avoidance of sudden stress and provision of an adequate diet should prevent the occurrence of resorption.

Miscarriage and abortion

Clinical signs: This occurs when the foetuses have reached a later stage in their development. If it occurs fairly early in gestation (up to around 40 days) the sow need not be systemically affected, and all that may be noticed is that she has traces of blood around her face acquired from cleaning herself. Later in gestation she is more likely to become noticeably ill; there may be severe blood loss at the same time, and this may prove fatal. It is, however, possible at any stage of gestation that only part of the litter is lost, and if the sow's condition improves it is possible that she can carry the rest of the litter to term and give birth normally.

Treatment: This may be unsuccessful if the sow is seriously ill. She must be placed in isolation. Supportive therapy, warmth and good food are necessary to maintain the pregnancy if only part of the litter is lost. An injection of vitamin B_{12} (Tx 48) may prove beneficial.

If there are any dead foetuses or placentas left inside the uterus, an injection of 1–2 iu oxytocin (Tx 41) can be given intramuscularly to aid their expulsion.

Comment: If a sow has had an abortion or miscarriage she must be rested and allowed to regain her strength for at least 2 months before being allowed to breed again. However, if the sow is in good condition despite having lost a litter at term she can either be used as a foster mother or put back with a boar to prevent her moping or becoming distressed whilst searching for her babies.

Abortions and premature births can also occur if the pregnant sow is penned with other nursing sows. As the pregnant sow takes interest in and cleans the other youngsters she may start having early contractions resulting in the loss of her litter. The placentas contain oxytocin and if ingested will trigger parturition. Parturition can be induced in this way from as early as the fifth week of gestation. It is therefore advisable to separate pregnant sows to prevent this problem.

High environmental temperatures have also been linked to an increased incidence of abortion. Sows that are exposed to a temperature of over 32°C (90°F) for an hour a day are at risk of losing their litters. It is very important to keep the caviary cool, especially during the hot summer months when most of the breeding takes place.

Abortion and resorption can occur as a consequence of a systemic infection and have been associated with *Bordetella bronchiseptica*, *Streptococcus pneumoniae* and *Salmonella* infections.

Toxoplasmosis

Guinea pigs may become infected with the protozoal parasite *Toxoplasma gondii*. The definitive host is the cat, and infection occurs when the guinea pig ingests food contaminated with cat faeces containing the oocyst stage of the parasite. Transmission is via the faecal–oral route or vertically through the placenta. Viable tissue cysts can persist in muscle, heart, eye and brain. Acute toxoplasmosis leads to vulval bleeding and abortion in pregnant sows.

Premature births

Clinical signs: The young are born small and weak, with short and very silky soft hair, and their nails are usually white. The sow will probably be unwell. Any birth which occurs before day 60 of gestation is premature. It occurs if the sow is in poor condition or is subject to a sudden stress. Premature births are also more common in sows that have been bred too young, i.e. sows under 5 months old.

Treatment: As long as the sow is not too weak she can be brought back to health with careful nursing and good feeding.

Intra-uterine haemorrhage

Clinical signs: The pregnant sow rapidly becomes unthrifty and she has a bloody discharge from the vulva.

Pathology: One or both horns of the gravid uterus will be full of blood, and the foetuses will be dead.

Comment: The aetiology of this condition is unknown, although it may be the result of a disorder of liver metabolism. Streptococcal infection has also been implicated.

Prevention: The animal must not be allowed to become obese as this will compromise liver function.

The hormonal maintenance of pregnancy

The successful initiation of pregnancy depends upon an extended secretion of luteal progesterone. The absolute requirement for progesterone persists throughout gestation, and a balance of both this hormone and oestrogen is necessary to maintain the pregnancy to full term. In many species these steroid hormones are provided by the ovarian corpus luteum, which is under higher control from the maternal pituitary, and removal of the ovaries or the pituitary leads to abortion. In the guinea pig, however, the pregnancy does not depend totally upon ovarian–pituitary interactions and these organs can be removed during the pregnancy without causing abortion. Experiments have shown that the pituitary is important for the first 3 days, and the ovaries for the first 28 days. Thereafter the majority of oestrogen and progesterone is synthesized in the placenta.

Comment: Stress and malnutrition in the first month will result in decreased activity of the ovaries, and it may be the result of insufficient hormone secretion by these under-functioning gonads that leads to early resorption.

Parturition

Parturition usually occurs 18–20 days after the first definite movements are felt. However, the actual onset of parturition is often difficult to predict, although there is sometimes evidence of nesting behaviour by the sow. There may also be subtle mood changes, probably associated with the pains of first stage labour. Before parturition the pubic ligaments begin to relax under the influence of the hormone relaxin, and the pubic symphyses start to separate. This process can happen up to a week before the onset of parturition, or it may occur as late as only 2 hours before. At the time of the birth this separation should be at least 15 mm, and is often as much as 22 mm.

The delivery of the young takes an average of 30 minutes, with an interval of 3–7 minutes between young. The majority of sows give birth at night.

Complications at parturition

Stillbirths

These account for the majority of losses in guinea pig breeding, and are usually the result of a long and difficult labour, and the young are found dead still in their amniotic sacs. There is evidence that feeding sows during gestation on pellets of over 20% protein is one of the factors which causes large foetuses that are stillborn.

Comment: The optimum age for a sow to have her first litter is at 5–6 months, and definitely before she is 10 months old. Between these ages her pelvic bones and muscles stretch easily to allow the passage of young through the birth canal, and this stretching remains permanent for subsequent litters. At 5 months old the pelvis is only partly fused, and fusion occurs over the next 5 months to produce a rigid structure. If the onset of breeding is delayed until the sow is over a year old the pelvic bones are already set and less flexible, and dystocia is more common.

Dystocia

This occurs when the young are too large to pass through the pelvic canal or if one of the foetuses is malpresented. Primary uterine inertia appears to be an uncommon cause of dystocia, although it may account for some sows close to parturition which are suddenly found dead in the morning despite seeming in good health previously.

Clinical signs: If a sow strains continually for over 20 minutes or fails to produce a young after 2 hours of intermittent straining, dystocia should be considered. If the sow remains in difficulties after this length of time she will rapidly become depressed and she may have a greenish–brown discharge from the vagina.

Careful examination of the cervix is necessary as is an assessment of the degree of separation of the pubic symphyses (which should be 15–20 mm).

Treatment: If there is adequate separation of the symphyses, parturition can be induced by injection of 1–2 units of oxytocin (Tx 41).

If part of a foetus is presented at the pelvic canal but appears stuck, plenty of lubrication (either Vaseline, liquid paraffin or obstetric lubricant) can be applied, and it may then be possible to deliver the foetus using gentle traction. Up to 10 ml of liquid paraffin can be introduced into the uterus via a short catheter or a piece of drip tubing attached to a syringe; this is especially useful if most of the natural lubrication provided by the maternal uterine fluids has been lost and the interior of the uterus has become dry.

Some difficult births, especially those in the breech position, can be helped by putting the sow's body under water to assist the contractions.

If parturition does not commence within 15 minutes of an oxytocin injection, or if the foetus is not delivered by other means, it will be necessary to proceed with caesarean section.

Comment: One of the major causes of dystocia is a foetal abnormality known as 'bull backed'. This usually arises when mating two roan-coloured guinea pigs together, because of the lethal gene carried by roans. The foetuses are massive and short-backed with the spine curved inwards, and the flesh along the back is open. The genitalia are displaced high on the rump, the legs are short and bent, and the head is large with the neck in extension. They are always born dead.

Roan × roan matings should be avoided as this lethal gene is also associated with microphthalmia and digestive disorders.

Prevention: Dystocia due to uterine inertia may be associated with a sub-clinical hypocalcaemia and calcium supplementation (Tx 46), once the pubic symphyses begin to separate, may prevent this problem.

Premature loss of amniotic fluid

This occurs very occasionally. A sow close to term will suddenly lose her large shape, even to the extent that she looks non-pregnant. This is due to early loss of the amniotic fluid which, if it does not immediately trigger parturition, will lead to foetal death. The sow will subsequently succumb to septicaemia.

Treatment: This is usually unsuccessful. The sow should be given a course of broad spectrum antibiotics.

Uterine prolapse

This can occur at parturition due to excessive straining, and is therefore often a sequel to dystocia, especially in the young sow. It has also been seen in an aged sow in very poor condition 2 weeks after parturition.

Treatment: This is usually unsuccessful. The uterus can be cleaned and replaced but it often reprolapses as soon as the sow strains to pass faeces. The guinea pig should be given an injection of 1–2 units of oxytocin (Tx 41) as the uterus is replaced. Affected sows are usually in too weak a state to survive surgery and euthanasia should be considered.

Vaginal prolapse

This is not a common condition, but some sows may have a permanent vaginal prolapse. Replacement is unsuccessful, and provided that the prolapse does not compromise the urethral opening it will not cause any problems. It is inadvisable to breed from sows with this condition as problems at parturition are unavoidable.

Post-partum haemorrhage

Some sows may bleed excessively after parturition. In the absence of trauma this has been linked to a vitamin K deficiency as it has been recorded in sows on a diet of dry food and poor hay only. Green foods are the major source of this vitamin and they must be included in the diet. The recommended requirement of vitamin K is 2 mg/kg of feed.

Treatment: Clinical cases are often fatal. Whatever the cause, an intramuscular injection of 0.5–1 mg/kg vitamin K (Konakion) can be tried, as this will aid blood clotting.

Mutilation of the young

Guinea pigs never eat their young deliberately. Injuries are only likely to occur during difficult births, especially those in the breech position when the sow may pull at a leg to assist delivery and inadvertantly mutilate the youngster.

Caesarean section

The sooner that dystocia is recognized and caesarean section is carried out, the better the chances are of survival of the sow and her litter. However, if the sow has already had a long and tiring labour and is depressed and weak, her chances of surviving an anaesthetic and surgery are much reduced. In cases where the sow is very weak the operation is best looked upon as a salvage procedure to deliver live young. Baby guinea pigs are born at a very advanced state of development, fully furred and with their eyes open, and hand-rearing is often very satisfying. They begin to nibble at solid food as early as their second day and can either be fostered or fed with a dropper (see later).

If, however, the dystocia is recognized early and caesarean section undertaken immediately it can be a successful and satisfying procedure. For details of the anaesthetics and preparation for surgery see Chapter 10.

Surgical procedure: The guinea pig is best placed in dorsal recumbency and the surgery carried out through a midline incision. The uterus should be opened close to its bifurcation, and the young and placentas delivered through this incision. This wound should then be closed using an inverting continuous suture of catgut or other absorbable material. Closure of the peritoneum and muscle can be done as one layer, preferably using an interrupted suture pattern. If possible, the preferred method of closing the skin is with a sub-cuticular continuous stitch using an absorbable suture (e.g. Vicryl), as the sow will not then have the added stress of returning to the surgery for suture removal, and it also produces a neat wound which does not interfere with the young as they sit under their mother or suckle from her.

Post-operatively the sow should be given an intramuscular injection of 1 unit of oxytocin (Tx 41), 10–15 ml of warmed glucose–saline given sub-cutaneously (Tx 15), and antibiosis only if the latter is considered necessary. Oral calcium supplementation (Tx 46) for the first 4–5 days after surgery will help prevent the development of post-operative ketosis (see section on pregnancy toxaemia). The sow should be allowed to recover quietly with her young in a warm box and offered glucose water to drink, either from a dish or a dropper. It may be necessary to give the young some supplementary hand-feeding if their mother is weak.

Comment: Sows that have had a caesarean section should not be bred from again as they carry a higher risk of developing complications at subsequent pregnancies.

Complications after parturition

Rejection of the young

Clinical signs: Some mothers, especially after they have experienced a difficult birth, appear terrified of their young and refuse to let them suckle, despite having initially licked them dry.

Treatment: Patient introduction of the young to the sow by gently holding them underneath her and letting her smell them. An intramuscular injection of 1 mg diazepam (Tx 44) will calm the sow and help her adjust to her babies. The sow is best penned in a small box covered with a towel with plenty of nourishing food near the babies whilst she learns to accept them.

Mastitis

Clinical signs: The affected gland may become warm, hard and swollen. In severe cases it may undergo ulceration and necrosis. The sow may become systemically ill.

Treatment: Broad spectrum antibiotics (Tx 1–9) for at least a week usually effect a cure. If ulceration is present, the gland must be kept clean and a topical agent such as Dermisol (Tx 23) can be used.

As the causal agents are numerous it may be advisable to run a culture test first so that an appropriate antibiotic can be chosen.

If the affected gland is very hard and painful, the application of hot compresses (cotton wool soaked in warm water) will be beneficial. If possible the mammary gland should be stripped frequently and the infected milk expressed. If the sow is fed no greens for a few days this will help decrease her milk production.

Comment: The factors which predispose to the development of this condition are usually environmental, i.e. a poor standard of cleanliness and a build up of faecal contamination in the hutch. It should therefore be possible to prevent its occurrence by improving hygiene and hutch cleanliness. Many bacteria have been isolated from these cases, especially *Pseudomonas aeruginosa*, *Pasturella multocida*, *Corynebacterium pyogenes*, *Staphylococcus aureus*, *Streptococcus* spp. and a variety of *Enterobacteriacae*.

Sore nipples

Clinical signs: This may occur if the sow is suckling a large litter. The teats may appear stretched and reddened, but not mastitic. It may also be a problem if the sow's milk supply is sparse, as the youngsters suck harder when they try to feed. The sow only has two inguinal mammary glands, and if she is nursing a large litter they are put under a lot of strain.

Treatment: Applying Kamillosan cream (Tx 24), a herbal preparation available from most chemists, several times a day to the affected area will soon relieve the soreness. It is perfectly safe to use this preparation whilst the young are suckling as it causes no harm on ingestion.

If the problem is due to agalactia or poor milk supply the sow can be provided with extra milk by giving her pellets or bran mash which has been soaked in milk, or by adding milk to her water bottle.

Comment: Occasionally a sow may possess two or three extra teats. However, these teats are generally blind and produce no milk.

Agalactia

Clinical signs: The young have a tucked-up starved appearance. The sow may resent the young suckling from her as her nipples may be sore. This problem is more common if the sow has had a long and difficult labour.

Treatment: Stress must be avoided as this inhibits the flow of milk. The sow and her young should be isolated and kept quiet. The young can be fed a milk preparation by dropper if necessary (see below). The sow can be offered a bran and brown bread mix soaked in milk, or alternatively her water bottle can be filled with evaporated milk diluted 1 : 1 with water. In 2–3 days her young will also be drinking from this bottle and the frequency of hand-supplementation can be reduced.

Injections of oxytocin soon after birth to improve milk let-down are not recommended as the stress they produce outweighs their beneficial effect.

Comment: Immediately after parturition, milk let-down is under the control of oxytocin which is released from the posterior pituitary following stimulation of the nipple during suckling and also from stimulus to the cervix as a foetus passes through the birth canal. The practice of eating the placentas is also a stimulus for milk production. For the remainder of lactation, milk secretion is under the control of prolactin, a hormone whose release is triggered by stimulation of the nipple during suckling. Therefore if the young are totally hand-reared it is unlikely that the sow will produce much milk as the stimulus for milk secretion is lost. However, if a sow is unstressed and well fed, her milk flow should return and it may only be necessary to supplement the young for the first 24 hours.

It is not necessary to hand-feed the young soon after birth as they may not become hungry for the first 12 hours, during which time the sow may have settled down and begun producing milk.

Eclampsia

Clinical signs: This is a rare condition but has been seen in older sows up to 7 days after parturition, especially if suckling a large litter. The sow becomes suddenly depressed and twitches. In later stages she goes into fits. Ketosis will also produce similar symptoms.

Treatment: An intraperitoneal injection of 5 ml of 10% calcium solution can be attempted, but it is unlikely to be successful in later stages of this condition.

Comment: During lactation, it is advisable to feed a variety of calcium-rich food. Carrots, beetroot and watercress are all good sources of calcium, although the latter must be fed sparingly. Sow thistle is also a useful supplement during lactation. Calcium supplementation (Tx 46) can be given to the sow during the last week of gestation and first week of lactation.

Skin complaints

Sows quite commonly develop raw patches on their rumps and ventral abdomens after birth. They may also develop a bare patch in the centre of their backs after parturition, known as a 'post-natal sore' (see Chapter 1). Hair loss is also common in the last trimester of pregnancy when the metabolic demands on the sow are high.

Orphans

As they are born at such an advanced stage of development, orphans have a good chance of survival. The young start picking at solid food and hay as early as the second day, and babies orphaned at 3 days old have been known to survive given no supplementation.

It is possible to use a foster mother if one is available; indeed, if two or more nursing females are penned together their young may steal feeds from the other mothers.

If no foster mother is available, the orphans can be reared on a suitable milk replacer fed through a dropper (e.g. Welpi or Sherley's Lactol). The powder should be mixed with water to a consistency that can run through a dropper, and initially they should be fed every 2 hours. They will probably take 1–2 ml of milk per feed during the first few days, and once they are 5 days old, and beginning to nibble at solid food, they need only be fed 4-hourly and at this stage they may take as much as 3 ml at one feed. However hand-feeding need not be started until the young are 12 hours old as they will not become hungry until then.

The milky mixture can also be mixed with brown bread in a dish so that they can learn to feed themselves. Minced carrot, beetroot and soaked pellets can also be offered in the early days, but they will soon nibble at adult food. If no foster mother with milk is available, it is a good idea to keep them with an adult guinea pig who can provide them with warmth and companionship. The baby guinea pigs will also copy the adult and soon start nibbling at solids. Once the young are drinking from the water bottle attached to the cage door this can be filled with evaporated milk diluted 1 : 1 with water.

As with the hand-rearing of any animal, care must be taken not to force the milk into the mouth in order to avoid causing inhalation pneumonia.

After each feed, it is important to clean their faces and to stimulate them to pass urine and faeces by stroking their lower abdomens with a piece of damp cotton wool.

An alternative recipe for a milk replacer that the author uses is evaporated milk diluted 1 : 2 with cooled boiled water and thickened with Farex to a consistency that will run through a dropper. A drop of (Tx 45) multivitamin drops available from the chemist, containing vitamins A, B, C and D- is added to one feed of the day. A probiotic such as Avipro (Tx 12) should also be added to each feed.

Comment: The composition of guinea pig milk is:

- 3.9% fat
- 8.1% protein
- 3% lactose

The composition of cows' milk is:

- 3.8% fat
- 3.3% protein
- 4.7% lactose

Thus evaporated milk is a close approximation, and as the young are soon nibbling at concentrates they can easily make up the protein deficit.

It is important to encourage the orphans to eat solid foods as early as possible because a high percentage of orphans which receive too much milk replacer develop cataracts and become blind. The development of cataracts is thought to be associated with the intake of too many complex sugars which are dissimilar to those found in natural guinea pig milk.

Hand-reared orphans may also develop skin conditions characterized by intense seborrhoea. This usually responds to shampooing with a human cradle cap shampoo.

Fostering

A suitable foster mother is one with a small litter of 2–3 days old. She should be put in a small box and her babies removed. The orphans should then be rubbed with the other young so that they all smell alike. Alternatively a mentholated vapour rub (e.g. Vick) can be dabbed under the mother's chin and on all the babies so that all different smells are eradicated. The orphans can then be introduced to the foster mother, and provided they are accepted the rest of the litter can be returned an hour later.

Nursing guinea pigs also make ideal foster parents for orphan chinchillas. The author has also successfully hand-reared a chinchilla with the help of a sow which had never had a litter, yet she instinctively took over every other aspect of caring for the orphan apart from the feeding.

INFERTILITY

The boar

Often it is the very large boars that are sterile. To check the boar, it is necessary to extrude his penis by pushing in on his abdomen just cranial to his genitalia. At the end of a normal penis there are two horns or prongs. These should be of equal length, but if one is missing or they are of differing lengths the boar will be sterile. Unfortunately some boars with normal looking genitalia can also be sterile.

If the boar is not given his first opportunity to mate before he is a year old, his sex drive will diminish rapidly. For this reason it is advisable to put a boar with his first sow when he is 4–5 months old. Overshowing will also lead to decreased sex drive.

Preputial prolapse

In adult boars the prepuce may stretch and this leads to the penis not being fully encased within the body, but up to 0.4 cm may be left outside and the prepuce falls into folds around it. Particles of food, hay and straw collect in the folds and cause irritation and infection. Such boars often become sterile.

Treatment: The penis and prepuce must be examined carefully, and if necessary cleaned with a weak saline solution (Tx 52) and topical anti-bacterial cream applied (e.g. Dermisol Tx 23). This must be applied sparingly as the boar is likely inadvertantly to ingest some when he collects his caecal faeces to redigest.

Preputial infections

These usually occur secondarily to foreign bodies such as grass seeds or sawdust becoming lodged in the prepuce. These may also lead to an inability to copulate. Preputial dermatitis may lead to a swelling of the prepuce and perineum.

Treatment: Removal of any foreign bodies and treatment of the infection. A topical preparation may be sufficient for this purpose (Tx 23–26).

Comment: Sawdust may also block the vagina of the female and lead to an inability of the male to achieve copulation. For this reason using sawdust as a bedding material should be discouraged, and the use of woodshavings recommended instead.

The sow

A sow may be naturally barren or she may become temporarily unable to conceive if she is in poor condition and underweight. A sow may become barren after a history of miscarriages or abortions. If she has recovered from an attack of cystitis she may also become infertile.

Many sows will just stop breeding once they reach 3–5 years of age. Cystic ovarian disease will also lead to infertility.

Treatment of both sexes

It is impossible to cure those that are naturally sterile, and these should be removed from the breeding programme.

(1) By improving the condition of the breeding sows their ability to conceive should return. It is important that litters are planned to coincide with maximum availability of greenstuff, i.e. March– September. It is therefore best to begin pairing the sows and boars in January.

(2) Each sow should be allowed adequate time to rest and regain her strength between litters (at least a month). No sow should have more than two or three litters a year.

(3) Addition of a little wheatgerm oil to the food daily may improve fertility. Wheatgerm consists almost entirely of vitamin E. A lack of adequate vitamin E leads to degeneration of the seminiferous tubules in the male.

(4) There should be adequate provision of good hay, as although the guinea pig does not build a nest it does like to burrow. Reproductive performance has been shown to decrease in the absence of hay.

(5) If the environmental temperature is too high this may lead to infertility. This phenomenon is seen during very hot summers. The recommendations for optimum temperature and humidity are:
- room temperature: 20–22°C (68–72°F)
- humidity: 45–65%

(6) It is important that the breeding hutches receive plenty of light. Both inadequate lighting and shortened daylight hours lead to infertility. 10–12 hours of daylight are required daily.

Comment: Guinea pigs are polyoestrus and come into season all the year round. At the time of ovulation the level of oestrogen in their serum rises to a maximum. Ovulation occurs when this coincides with a surge of a second hormone, luteinizing hormone (LH). The latter is released from the anterior pituitary under the control of GnRH (gonadotrophin-releasing factor) from the hypothalamus. The LH surge is subject to control by a daily rhythm. The GnRH neurones are influenced by a neural signal carrying information about light/dark cycles from the retina. Thus, if the breeding stock are kept in poor light there will be insufficient stimulus for this sequence of hormone release and therefore no trigger for ovulation.

Therefore, by improving the lighting to the breeding quarters and, if necessary, using artificial lighting to create the required 10–12 hours of light per day, it should be possible to provide the correct environmental stimuli necessary for this sequence of hormonal events leading to ovulation.

The hormonal control of gonadal activity in the male is constant, and not cyclical as in the female. However, environmental factors play just as important a role in governing the reproductive activity of the male, and thus the above comments about infertility apply equally to both sexes.

It is best not to breed from sows or boars which take a long time to mate successfully as their offspring are likely to inherit the same problems.

Cystic ovaries

The incidence of this condition in guinea pigs is unknown but is thought to be quite high. It may be an important contributing factor to sow infertility or her inability to carry a litter to term.

The ovary can contain multiple fluid-filled cysts up to 3 cm in diameter, and the condition is usually bilateral. The guinea pig may have bilateral hair loss over its flanks.

Treatment: Ovariohysterectomy. Alternatively the cysts can be drained via percutaneous needle aspiration.

Metritis

Mild cases may only result in a failure to become pregnant. More severe cases may occur after abortion or difficult births and are usually fatal. Some cases have been associated with *Bordetella* infection.

Vaginal discharge

This must not be confused with the normal opaque creamy coloured urine which may be seen by the genitalia. A vaginal discharge accompanied by infertility is suggestive of metritis.

Treatment: A vaginal swab should be taken for culture and sensitivity tests. A suitable broad-spectrum antibiotic can then be used to treat the infection (Tx 1–9).

Comment: Haemolytic streptococci are commonly implicated as a cause of this condition.

Cystic endometritis

Clinical signs: The sow passes blood from her vulva, initially inter-mittently, but as the condition progresses the bleeding may become profuse. The haematuria is not accompanied by dysuria (a feature of cystitis and urolithiasis).

Treatment: The guinea pig should be radiographed to eliminate uro-lithiasis from the differential diagnosis. Ovariohysterectomy is curative.

Castration

The inguinal canal of the male guinea pig remains open throughout life, and there is therefore an increased risk of a prolapse of abdominal contents after castration. In times of stress (e.g. anaesthesia) the male guinea pig is able to withdraw his testes completely into the abdomen. Castration can be performed from 12 weeks of age, or when the guinea pig has reached 650 g body weight.

Surgical procedure: A skin incision should be made in the scrotum directly over each testis. The tunic should then be incised and the testis can be grasped. Gentle traction will reveal the spermatic cord and a mass of fat. The epididymis is separated from the gubernaculum. The spermatic cord and spermatic blood vessels should be ligated below the testis. The fat should be preserved, as its presence will help block the inguinal canal after surgery and reduce the risk of herniation. Once the testis is removed the tunic should be closed, and this will effectively block the inguinal canal. If it is not possible to close the tunic, the skin incision should be extended cranially and the inguinal ring closed to prevent post-operative herniation. The skin can be closed with an absorbable suture, with either simple interrupted sutures, or a continuous sub-cuticular suture.

Ovariohysterectomy

Ovariohysterectomy can be performed in cases of cystic ovaries, cystic endometritis, or following caesarean section.

Surgical procedure: Ovariohysterectomy is performed through a midline incision, and the uterus removed after ligating the ovarian blood vessels and those at the cervix. The peritoneum should be closed using a mono-filament non-absorbable suture to reduce the risk of post-operative her-niation. The skin can be closed with a sub-cuticular suture or a continuous apposition suture to prevent suture removal by the patient. Before final closure of the peritoneum 10–15 ml of warmed glucose–saline (Tx 15) can be given by intraperitoneal injection. Some analgesia should be given at the time of surgery.

Neoplasia

Mammary gland neoplasia

Tumours of the mammary glands can occur in both sexes, and are often unilateral. The majority are benign fibroadenomas. Malignant adeno-carcinomas are seen less frequently; these are locally invasive, but rarely metastasize.

Treatment: The tumour should be removed with a wide margin of normal tissue. As the two inguinal mammary glands do not share a common blood or lymphatic supply, only the affected gland need be removed. The skin can be sutured using a mattress suture (if it is under tension), or a continuous interlocking suture. An Elizabethan collar may be necessary to prevent the guinea pig interfering with the wound.

3 THE URINARY SYSTEM

ANATOMY

The guinea pig has two kidneys, the right kidney being placed further forward in the body than the left. A ureter runs from each renal pelvis to enter the bladder (see Fig. 3.1). A single urethra runs from the bladder to the urethral opening.

The male urethra is longer and less distendable than that of the female and as it passes from the bladder to the urethral opening it is closely associated with the vesicular (coagulating) gland, the prostate and the bulbourethral gland.

PHYSIOLOGY

Normal guinea pig urine is opaque and creamy yellow in colour. It is alkaline and has a normal pH of 9. The urine occasionally contains crystals of ammonium phosphate and calcium carbonate. This crystaluria accounts for a build up of scale in the hutches which can easily be removed by cleaning with a weak acid solution.

Urinary tract disorders

Little is known about the incidence of kidney disease in guinea pigs and many definitive diagnoses are only made at post-mortem. However, symptoms of lower urinary tract disorders are more frequently seen in general practice.

Fig. 3.1 The urinary tract (showing position of male accessory glands).

SYMPTOMS OF URINARY TRACT DISORDERS

Polydipsia

The average water intake of a guinea pig is 10 ml/100 g. However, this is very variable, and if the diet consists of foods with a high water content, e.g. lettuce and other succulent green foods, very little extra water will be drunk. Water intake does increase by varying amounts during pregnancy and lactation.

Polydipsia can be expected to occur in cases of chronic renal failure and diabetes. Polydipsia accompanied by a large abdominal swelling has been seen in a case of hydronephrosis of both kidneys. The affected individual was not ill but was euthanased when the swelling became severe.

A diet consisting of a large amount of dandelions, which induce diuresis, will lead to a resultant transient polydipsia.

Polyuria

The average urinary output of an adult is 20–25 ml per day. Polyuria is only seen as a consequence of polydipsia, or when eating large quantities of foods with diuretic properties (e.g. dandelions). Excess urine output may lead to urine scalding which can present a problem in both sexes, and this is seen clinically as a moist dermatitis around the genitals ventrally in the sow, and around the rump in the male.

This consequent urine scalding can be treated with topical applications of Dermisol or Vetsovate twice daily (Tx 23 or 26). The affected area can be protected with Vaseline or a resistant barrier cream such as zinc and castor oil cream.

Guinea pigs which are prone to the development of this condition should be kept on an absorbent bedding such as newspaper and woodshavings to minimize the problem of urine soaking their coats.

Haematuria ('bloody urine')

Passing blood in the urine is a fairly common complaint, and is seen equally frequently in boars and sows.

Clinical signs: The affected animal is often still in good health, or may exhibit pain during urination, by arching its back and crying.

Causes of haematuria: These include:

(1) Cystitis. If cystitis is suspected a course of broad-spectrum antibiotics can be given for 7 days; ones that are commonly used are enro-floxacin or trimethoprim (Tx 1 and 9). A human preparation of nitrofurantoin (Tx 6) has also been successful at a dose of 50 mg a day for 3 days.

   Once a sow has had an attack of cystitis she may become infertile.

(2) Neoplasia. Unfortunately the passing of bloody urine is frequently associated with tumours of the bladder or uterus. If the guinea pig is still bright, eating and not in severe discomfort, supportive measures can be instituted (B vitamins and iron-rich foods such as spinach, grass and dandelions). If there is severe discomfort euthanasia is the kindest option.

(3) Urolithiasis. See below.

(4) Cystic endometritis.

True haematuria must be differentiated from the red-coloured urine produced by guinea pigs on a diet consisting of large quantities of beetroot.

Crystaluria

The urine is naturally alkaline and may contain phosphate and carbonate crystals. These generally cause no problems, but may form as a scale around the cage. However, together with other predisposing factors such as low water intake, these crystals may form larger calculi.

Occlusion of the penile urethra

Coagulum from the vesicular glands may block the terminal portion of the urethra and lead to a secondary cystitis.

Clinical signs: Pain on urination is a common feature. Haematuria associated with the secondary cystitis may also be evident.

Treatment: Cleansing of the affected area, and broad-spectrum antibiotics if there is a concurrent cystitis (Tx 1–9).

Urolithiasis

The formation of stones is more common in the boar as his urethra is longer and less distendable than that of the sow. Males also possess an os penis. Normal urine may contain small calculi and under certain circumstances these may form larger stones. In older males, concretions are found in the urethra and in the prepuce, and these in part are the result of congealed ejaculum and crystals which readily become infected with *Pseudomonas aeruginosa*, *Proteus* and *Escherichia coli*.

If just a few stones are present in the urinary tract they may only partially obstruct the urinary flow, and over a period of time the resultant back pressure on the kidneys may cause a progressive hydronephrosis.

Clinical signs: These are variable. In mild cases they may be absent, whilst more severely affected individuals may exhibit dysuria or anuria (seen as a hunched posture and crying when attempting to urinate), haematuria, anorexia and listlessness.

The stones may be palpable and occasionally they can be felt as a hard lump inside the prepuce. They will also be evident on radiographs.

Treatment: (1) Surgical removal from the bladder and subsequent antibiotic treatment has been reported to be successful. (2) Stones present inside the sheath can be removed manually by extruding the penis. (3) Small calculi may be dissolved if the urine is acidified; however, guinea pigs do have difficulty in removing an acid load. Some acidification of the urine can be achieved by feeding more of foods with a high acid content, e.g. apple and beetroot. High doses of vitamin C (100 mg/day) can also be used to acidify the urine.

Comment: The aetiology of stone formation is unclear. However, predisposing factors include a low water intake, nutritional imbalances and bacterial infections. Diets that have a high calcium content (those containing alfalfa) and a high vitamin D content make stone formation most likely. There also seems to be an inherited disposition to their development.

Hydronephrosis

One or both kidneys may become cystic and fluid-filled.

Clinical signs: Polydipsia and palpable abdominal swellings. In the early stages, the guinea pig remains well, but as the condition progresses other signs associated with chronic renal failure become apparent. This condition is usually seen in guinea pigs over the age of 4 years.

Pathology: The affected kidney has most of its normal structure replaced and becomes a fluid-filled sac with a rim of atrophied parenchyma. When a single kidney becomes hydronephrotic the other kidney can function alone. However, chronic renal failure will occur if the other kidney also becomes affected. Thus in post-mortem examinations the condition is often found to be bilateral.

Acute renal failure

This is an infrequent but fatal condition in guinea pigs. However, it may occur due to oxalic acid poisoning which may result from the ingestion of large amounts of beetroot, spinach or dock leaves once the stems have turned woody, as all of these contain oxalic acid.

Clinical signs before death include depression, salivation and muscle tremors. Numerous crystals of calcium oxalate precipitate out in the kidney and urinary tract.

Chronic renal failure

Clinical signs: Chronic renal disease is insidious in onset and initially the only sign may be polydipsia. As the disease progresses there may be a period of anorexia and depression, diarrhoea, then collapse and death.

Pathology: The affected kidneys are smaller in size, and much of their parenchyma is replaced with fibrous tissue ('end-stage' kidneys). If the renal failure is as a result of progressive hydronephrosis, the normal parenchyma will be replaced by a thin-walled sac which will be full of fluid.

Comment: Staphylococcal pododermatitis may progress to renal amyloidosis and nephritis. Chronic interstitial nephritis may also be seen as a consequence of diabetes and its associated hyperglycaemia.

Diabetes

Clinical signs: Diabetes is common in guinea pigs. Polydipsia and weight loss occur despite the guinea pig maintaining a good appetite. Some individuals may also develop cataracts. Glycosuria may also predispose to cystitis.

Diagnosis: Blood glucose can be determined from a drop of blood obtained by overclipping a toenail. Normal values lie between 60 and 125 mg/100 ml (3–7 mmol/litre).

Comment: Exogenous insulin is not required for survival, and spontaneous remissions are common.

4 THE RESPIRATORY SYSTEM

ANATOMY AND PHYSIOLOGY

Guinea pigs possess a normal mammalian respiratory system with no specific peculiarities. The healthy guinea pig will only breathe through its nose and therefore mouth breathing is a sign of respiratory distress.

SYMPTOMS OF RESPIRATORY DISORDERS

Sneezing

All guinea pigs sneeze occasionally, especially if they are exposed to dusty food or hay. Guinea pigs bedded on fine sawdust are also inclined to sneeze frequently. Sneezing is their body's natural defence mechanism for keeping their nasal passages clear. However, if the sneezing becomes more frequent or it is accompanied by a mucopurulent or haemopurulent discharge it may be a symptom of a more serious disease condition.

Epistaxis

Bleeding from the nose may be a symptom of vitamin K deficiency. This can arise if the diet consists of dry food and poor hay only, as the major source of this vitamin is from greenstuffs.

Epistaxis may also be present after trauma, especially if the guinea pig has fallen on its head.

Nasal discharge

A mucopurulent discharge is usually a symptom of upper or lower respiratory tract infection. However, this must not be confused with a normal milky fluid which is occasionally exuded from the nose and eyes as part of the natural grooming process.

Coughing

As with sneezing, all guinea pigs will cough occasionally, and this need not be related to a pathological condition but is assumed to be a part of the body's natural defence mechanism.

Snuffles

Certain types of guinea pig, especially those with short noses, may snuffle as they breathe. This problem may be present from birth and these youngsters are more prone to developing respiratory disease later. These guinea pigs encounter similar problems to those of the brachycephalic breeds of dog.

Ruttling

This term describes a rough sounding wheezy type of breathing made by guinea pigs (râles). It is often a symptom of an infectious disease condition; however, it may present unassociated with a disease process. The origin of this sound is unclear.

RESPIRATORY INFECTIONS

Predisposing factors: A change in environmental temperature, humidity or ventilation. Ammonia produced as a consequence of a build up of dirty litter will also weaken the resistance of the respiratory tract to infection. Other factors include a sudden diet change, diets low in vitamin C and overcrowding. The young, old and pregnant are the most susceptible groups for developing respiratory disease.

Pneumonia

Clinical signs: The symptoms of pneumonia are similar regardless of the causative agent and include dyspnoea, ruttling, sneezing accompanied by a nasal discharge and coughing. The affected guinea pig adopts a tucked-up appearance, becomes depressed and anorexic and, if left untreated, will die. In some cases the infection progresses to the middle and inner ear causing torticollis. Even with treatment the outcome can be fatal.

This condition can be caused by numerous bacterial and viral agents. The most common of these is *Bordetella bronchiseptica*, but others include *Streptococcus zooepidemicus* (see Chapter 7), *Streptococcus pneumoniae*, *Klebsiella pneumoniae*, *Pseudomonas aeruginosa* and *Pasturella* spp.

Bordetella and *Streptococcus pneumoniae* may also cause uterine infections and abortion, either as a separate entity or as part of a more generalized infection.

Diagnosis: Isolation of the causal agent from a culture of tracheal exudate.

Pathology: At post-mortem, *Bordetella* infections reveal consolidation of a lobe of lung, accompanied by signs of a purulent bronchitis, suppuration, exudation and haemorrhage. *Streptococcus* infections produce seropurulent and fibrinopurulent lesions of the pleural cavity, lungs, pericardium and occasionally the peritoneum. In cases of sudden death in pregnant sows, abscesses may be present in the uterine wall.

Treatment: Broad-spectrum antibiotics, e.g. a trimethoprim sulphona-mide combination (Tx 9) or enrofloxacin (Tx 1). However, antibiotics may not eliminate the carrier state. In the case of *Streptococcus zooepidemi-cus* the use of a cephalosporin (Tx 2) is recommended. If the lungs are very congested concurrent treatment with a diuretic (e.g. frusemide – Lasix 5% solution – at a dose rate of 0.1 ml given by intramuscular injection) is recommended.

The affected guinea pig must be isolated in a warm, clean and well-ventilated environment. A little mentholated vapour rub (e.g. Vick) can be applied around the hutch and this will help clear the nasal passages. Alternatively eucalyptus oil can be used for the same purpose. Some Vick can also be dabbed on the chest or on the inside of the forelegs where the skin is bare. If the guinea pig is anorexic, an appetite stimulant such as Vetrumex (Tx 13) can be given mixed with some water and 2–3 drops of multivitamins (Tx 45). An old remedy for colds and asthma was to feed coltsfoot, and if this is available it can be included in the guinea pig's diet.

Increasing the water vapour content of the environment by using the steam from a boiling kettle, or by placing the individual in the bathroom will help soothe the nasal passages and loosen the mucus in the bronchi.

Epidemiology: This may include the following conditions:

(1) *Bordetella bronchiseptica* may be introduced via symptomless carriers of other species, e.g. dogs, cats and rabbits, and care must be taken if these species are brought into close contact with guinea pigs. Outbreaks of *Bordetella* are precipitated by stress. The incubation period is 3–7 days.

(2) *Streptococcus pneumoniae* is spread by direct or indirect (aerosol) routes. Some individuals may exist as symptomless carriers and carry the organism in their upper respiratory tract.

Prevention: The environmental factors should be kept constant. Where possible the room temperature should be 20–22°C, and the relative humidity 45–65%. The hutches should be cleaned regularly to prevent the accumulation of ammonia. The ventilation should be good, but the caviary must be free from draughts.

Vaccination using an autogenous formalin killed bacterin given intramuscularly has been described. 0.2 ml of a porcine bordetellosis vaccine was given, and repeated 2–3 weeks later. This gives adequate protection for 4–6 months, and its use was successful in eliminating the carrier state from an affected colony. Porcine *Bordetella* bacterins will also protect guinea pigs against fatal pneumonias. Vaccines must not contain aluminium hydroxide as guinea pigs may react to it.

Several drops (one drop in each nostril) of a canine intranasal vaccine may provide similar protection against *Bordetella*.

Adenovirus

This is described separately as it does not require a bacterial co-pathogen to cause respiratory disease, and in certain circumstances it can be fatal.

The incubation period is 5–10 days. Infection may be inapparent; however, in stressed or immunodeficient guinea pigs (neonates, weanlings and aged animals) it can cause a severe pneumonia.

Diagnosis: Histopathology will demonstrate a bronchitis and bronchiolitis with typical intranuclear inclusion bodies.

Treatment: Supportive therapy. Antibiotics to prevent any secondary bacterial infection.

Mycoplasma

Mycoplasma caviae colonises the nasopharynx and the vagina. It does not cause clinical disease on its own, and is not thought to be pathogenic.

Non-infectious ruttling

The aetiology of this is unclear. Guinea pigs of the short-nosed type seem more prone to developing abnormal respiratory sounds. It is more common in winter when the hay and dry food are more dusty. Other causes that have been suggested are sawdust, high pollen counts, and stress in highly strung individuals. In the cases associated with hay and pollen the likely mechanism is the development of an allergic type bronchitis, which may clear once the allergen has been eliminated.

This condition has also been referred to as 'beetroot ruttle' in the past but no link between the two has been made.

Clinical signs: The respiratory sounds become wheezy and rough sounding. In comparison with infectious conditions the guinea pig remains otherwise healthy and eats well.

Treatment: A 5-day course of sulphadimidine (Tx 7) can be given, but some cases may never be completely cured.

5 THE DIGESTIVE SYSTEM

ANATOMY

The anatomy of the digestive tract is displayed in Fig. 5.1. In contrast to other rodents the guinea pig has a very long colon, which accounts for 60% of the length of its intestines. It also has a large caecum for digestion of cellulose, a feature which is typical of a herbivore. The wall of this organ is thin and it contains numerous lateral pouches which further increase its capacity, with the result that the caecum is able to contain up to 65% of the gastrointestinal contents at any one time.

The stomach is non-glandular and the spleen is closely associated to it and is relatively broad. The female's spleen is significantly larger and heavier than that of the male.

PHYSIOLOGY

The intestinal tract contains large numbers of non-pathogenic protozoa, and *Candida albicans* is also present in normal gut flora. The bacterial component of normal gastrointestinal flora is made up of a majority of Gram-positive anaerobic cocci and *Lactobacilli*. Gram-negative *Escherichia coli* and *Clostridia* are absent from the normal flora or are present only in very small amounts.

The process of digestion may take anything from 5 hours to several days; the average gastrointestinal transit time is between 13 and 30 hours. The guinea pig, typical of a herbivore, spends a large proportion of each day eating. The average food consumption is 6 g/100 g of body weight, and up to 75% of the food intake may be in the form of concentrates. The average water intake is 85 ml for an adult, but this figure is very variable depending upon the amount of moist green food consumed.

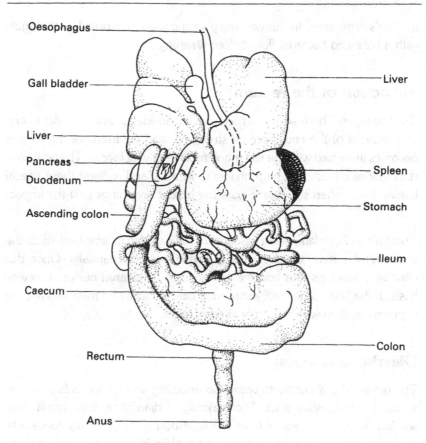

Oesophagus

Gall bladder

Liver

Liver

Pancreas

Duodenum

Ascending colon

Caecum

Rectum

Anus

Spleen

Stomach

Ileum

Colon

Fig. 5.1 The digestive tract.

Guinea pigs are very fastidious in their eating habits and do not accommodate alterations easily. If the composition of their diet is altered suddenly they may just stop eating and starve to death. Similarly if their water supply is changed from a bowl to a water bottle or vice versa they may suffer water deprivation until they adjust to using the new source of water.

Coprophagia

The eating of its own droppings is a normal part of the digestive process. The guinea pig selectively eats the smaller moist droppings taking them directly from the anus. These lighter and softer faeces are caecal faeces and contain the important B-complex vitamins which are formed by bacterial flora in the caecum. By redigesting these faeces the guinea pig satisfies its need for B vitamins. Young guinea pigs will also be seen eating their mother's droppings. In this way the young guinea pigs populate their guts with a balanced bacterial flora before weaning.

Impaction of the rectum

Clinical signs: This is seen as a hard swelling inside the anus of older boars. The muscles of the anus become stretched, and the inside of the rectum becomes impacted with the softer and moister caecal faeces. The boar may start to lose condition if he is unable to remove and re-digest these caecal faeces. He is often still able to pass the harder droppings past the impaction.

Treatment: Petroleum jelly (Vaseline) or olive oil can be smeared inside the anus and the mass of faeces can be squeezed out manually. Once this condition develops in a boar he will need to be cleared out on a weekly basis. If the boar is not redigesting any caecal faeces he may also require supplementation with a vitamin B complex.

Diarrhoea (scours)

The guinea pig is unable to vomit, so anything that it ingests has to pass through the digestive tract. The majority of diarrhoea cases result from sudden dietary changes or from the ingestion of poor quality foodstuffs. However, if it is seen as an enzootic problem infectious causes must be considered. It is also seen as a symptom in more generalized disease conditions such as chronic kidney or liver failure.

Infectious causes of diarrhoea

Salmonella

The causal agents are usually *Salmonella typhimurium* or *Salmonella enteriditis*. The disease generally enters the caviary via carrier mice and rats which may contaminate the food and hay.

Clinical signs: Acute enteritis which may be haemorrhagic; also sudden deaths (septicaemia), abortions, and in chronic cases weight loss and poor condition. The disease will spread rapidly through the caviary.

Pathology: At post-mortem there is splenic enlargement and focal necrosis of this organ and the liver which may also be enlarged. There will also be hyperaemia of the intestines accompanied by mesenteric lymph node enlargement. In per-acute cases splenic enlargement may be the only feature, and there are no lesions in carrier animals.

Diagnosis: Isolation of *Salmonella* spp. in faecal samples.

Treatment: Affected animals should be destroyed and preferably disposed of by burning as *Salmonella* is zoonotic. Healthy guinea pigs should be removed from the affected premises and housed separately elsewhere. All premises and feeding and drinking utensils should be thoroughly disinfected, and any bedding and hay should be burnt.

Chloramphenicol (Tx 3) at a dose of 20–55 mg/kg orally three times a day or 6.5 mg/kg injected intramuscularly twice daily will effect some cures, but its use is very likely to produce resistant strains and perpetuate the carrier state which is an undesirable consequence.

Comment: Chronic cases and those which recover are likely to become carriers of *Salmonella* and they should also be destroyed to prevent further outbreaks of this disease.

Considering the public health risk of this disease, it is recommended to depopulate the caviary completely rather than risk perpetuating the disease in its carrier state.

Yersinia (pseudotuberculosis)

Clinical signs: Both acute and chronic forms of this disease are recognized. The acute form causes septicaemia and death within 48 hours. The more chronic form causes a longer period of diarrhoea and weight loss, and occasionally dysponea and coughing, often culminating in death after 3–4 weeks. During this period, any young of the affected guinea pig may become congenitally or neonatally affected. In an emaciated guinea pig the enlarged mesenteric lymph nodes can often be palpated through the abdomen.

In some cases the infection may be contained in the cervical lymph nodes, and this must be differentiated from abscesses and cervical lymphadenitis (see Chapters 1 and 7). In such cases the condition is not usually fatal.

Diagnosis: Culture of *Yersinia pseudotuberculosis* from blood or lymph nodes. The organism can also be cultured from faecal samples.

Pathology: Nodular, caseous lesions in the mesenteric lymph nodes, and focal necrosis of the liver and spleen. There may also be lesions in the lungs and pleura.

Treatment: Like *Salmonella*, the condition is zoonotic. Because of this, and the likelihood of post-treatment carriers, culling is the only effective control measure. Regular abdominal palpation of the mesenteric lymph nodes will help in detecting asymptomatic carriers. Wild birds and rodents must be excluded from the food storage area.

Comment: The disease is transmitted to guinea pigs via wild birds and rodents which contaminate their green foods. Any green foods should be washed before being fed to guinea pigs. Once it is endemic in a breeding population more chronic forms are seen, and in some cases the infection is passed vertically in the milk. *Yersinia* is also present in dust, soil and water.

Clostridia

Clostridia spp. are normally present in small numbers in the large intestine. In certain circumstances (e.g. during antibiotic administration) they are able to proliferate and cause a fatal enterotoxaemia.

Clinical signs: An acute onset of profuse diarrhoea, either green-brown or watery, accompanied by other signs of depression, bloat, abdominal pain and a fetid odour.

Diagnosis: At post-mortem there are signs of a haemorrhagic enteritis, and the gut lumen contains green-brown mucoid material.

Clostridial species can be cultured from the lumen of affected portions of intestine.

Treatment: None available – the condition is fatal.

Escherichia coli

Escherichia coli is not a normal inhabitant of the gastrointestinal tract, and if it is isolated in large numbers from a case of enteritis it is usually significant.

Clinical signs: Anorexia, listlessness, salivation, diarrhoea with mucus and blood, followed by shock and death within 48 hours. Per-acute cases may present as sudden death, and in chronic cases rectal prolapse may follow the initial diarrhoea. There may be up to 85% mortality in a stud. The clinical signs resemble 'watery mouth' syndrome in lambs, which is also caused by E. coli.

Diagnosis: Diagnosis is at post-mortem. In per-acute (sudden death) cases there may be fluid in the chest from which E. coli may be cultured. In acute cases there are caecal haemorrhages, and E. coli may be cultured from the caecal wall, and the heart blood. Caecal haemorrhages are present in chronic cases.

Treatment: This is directed at correcting the ketosis, and counteracting the endotoxaemia. Dexamethasone can be given to correct the ketosis, and flunixine megulamine can be given daily for 3 days to combat endotoxic shock. Fluids are extremely important, and an oral rehydration preparation should be given regularly. A probiotic should also be administered. An antibiotic such as enrofloxacin can be given at a dose of 5 mg/kg daily.

Comment: E. coli is generally only thought to be an environmental pathogen causing clinical disease when hygiene is poor. However, outbreaks of E. coli diarrhoea in well managed studs suggest that it can be a primary pathogen. Attention to hygiene is very important, as is a good diet in preventing such outbreaks. Sub-clinical vitamin C deficiency can predispose the gastrointestinal system to infection, and it is important to ensure that there is enough vitamin C in the diet.

Enteropathies of unknown origin

A per-acute necrosis of the mucosa of the caecum and large intestine leading to sudden death has been reported.

Parasitic causes of diarrhoea

Parasitic enteritis is rarely a problem in guinea pigs.

Nematodes

The only nematode which affects guinea pigs is *Paraspidodera uncinata* and infection is generally associated with guinea pigs housed in outdoor runs. Heavy infestations may cause enteritis. *Paraspidodera* usually resides in the caecum and the adult is 11–28 mm long.

Treatment: Fenbendazole at a rate of 100 mg/kg given orally or piperazine (Tx 33) at a dilution of 3 mg/ml in the drinking water.

Protozoa

A large number of protozoa can be carried, but these are not usually pathogenic with the exception of *Coccidia* (see below). Of the non-pathogenic species *Trichomonas* and *Entamoeba* spp. are the most frequently isolated.

Complications due to these organisms are generally associated with poor husbandry or severe debilitation from other causes. Sporadic deaths preceded by a short period (3–8 hours) of diarrhoea have been seen in association with a large burden of *Trichomonas* spp. in guinea pigs housed on deep straw litter.

Treatment: Metronidazole (Tx 32, Flagyl) at a dose of 20 mg/kg diluted in the drinking water for 10 days.

Cestoda

Infection due to *Cestoda* is also very infrequent, but the guinea pig may act as an alternative host to *Cestoda* which normally use other rodents as their hosts, such as *Hymenolepis* spp., *Taenia crassicollis* and *Echinococcus granulosus*.

Heavy infestation by these tapeworms may cause enteritis, intestinal obstruction or retarded growth.

Treatment: Praziquantel (Tx 34, Droncit, Bayer) at a dose of 5–10 mg/kg orally or 5 mg/kg by subcutaneous injection.

Cryptosporidium

This has been implicated as a cause of diarrhoea, weight loss and death in young animals, but is unlikely to be a problem unless the guinea pig is immunocompromised.

Coccidiosis

Eimeria caviae is the coccidial species recognized in guinea pigs, and infection is usually contracted by the ingestion of contaminated food. It is, however, a very infrequent problem in the domestic guinea pig.

Guinea pigs may become infected with other *Coccidia* spp. if they are in contact with rabbits.

Clinical signs: The droppings are slimy in appearance and contain blood. Affected individuals look generally unthrifty and youngsters fail to gain weight.

Diagnosis: Oocysts are present in the faeces and they may be seen on microscopic examination of the supernatant layer of faecal matter after flotation, or on examination of a wet mount prepared directly from the intestinal contents.

Pathology: At post-mortem petechial haemorrhages and greyish-white nodules are present in the wall of the colon.

Treatment: Sulphadimidine (Tx 35) is given to affected guinea pigs for 5 days. Cleanliness is essential and if possible the guinea pigs should be housed on wire flooring to prevent the incidence of reinfection. Oocysts which are present in the hutch can be destroyed by cleaning with a 1% ammonia solution.

Comment: The presence of oocysts of *Eimeria caviae* does not necessarily mean that it is the primary pathogen in a case of diarrhoea.

Ascaridae

Ascaridae are not a natural parasite of guinea pigs, but they may occur if the guinea pig is grazing on grass which has been contaminated with dog or cat faeces.

Clinical signs: Weight loss and unthriftiness, diarrhoea and occasionally signs of intestinal obstruction.

Treatment: Oral administration of fenbendazole at a dose rate of 100 mg/kg as a single dose.

Non-infectious causes of diarrhoea

Dietary

This is a relatively common cause of diarrhoea which affects individuals in the caviary rather than causing a disease of zoonotic proportions.

Sudden change of diet: This often occurs in spring when there is a sudden increase in the availability of greenstuffs and the temptation is to overfeed rather than to reintroduce green foods slowly and carefully.

Grass clippings: These are one of the major offenders for causing scours as they rapidly overheat. They should only be fed immediately after they have been cut and any that are uneaten after a few hours should be removed.

Plants with a laxative action: If large quantities of these green foods are fed together this will result in diarrhoea. Such plants include groundsel and dandelions. They should be fed in balance with plants with an astringent action such as shepherd's purse, bramble leaves and young dock leaves.

Mouldy or frosted food: Care must be taken when collecting wild greens from the hedgerows, especially in late summer, to ensure that there is no white mould on the underside of the leaves, as this will cause a mucoid enteritis.

Roots must be completely thawed before they are fed if they have been picked when the ground is frozen, and greens covered in frost should not be fed.

Similarly, food which has been taken from the refrigerator should not be fed immediately, but allowed to warm a little first. Fresh food remaining in the hutch at night should be removed during the cold weather as it is likely to freeze overnight.

The feeding of frosted food will damage the lining of the stomach wall causing ulceration and subsequent diarrhoea.

Mouldy hay may contain fungal species, notably *Absidia ramosa* and *A. corymbifera*. These may cause a transient localized reaction in the mesenteric lymph nodes and often a profuse diarrhoea. The fungi may also colonize other organs such as the kidneys and spleen with fatal consequences.

Cereals, particularly maize, may become contaminated with fungal spores of *Aspergillus flavus*, and ingestion of these will cause a fatal aphlatoxicosis.

Clinical signs: Although the droppings are loose, the guinea pig is still bright in the early stages, and usually continues to eat normally. If the condition is allowed to progress unattended the guinea pig may become dull, depressed and anorexic.

Treatment: All green food must be removed from the diet and the guinea pig fed solely on good hay and dry food. Astringents such as bramble leaves (with the thorns removed) and shepherd's purse can be fed. Arrowroot, either as crumbled biscuits or in its dry form mixed with water, is another useful astringent.

Some breeders recommend feeding a bran mash soaked in water to which a little vitamin C has been added instead of the dry food. If the guinea pig's normal diet includes a molasses-enriched dry mix this should certainly be replaced with bran as the molasses will perpetuate the diarrhoea. Plenty of water should be given, and in some instances giving diluted liquid Lectade (Tx 16) will be beneficial.

If the affected animal is severely dehydrated the subcutaneous administration of warmed glucose–saline (Tx 15) or electrolyte solution (Hartmann's) may be beneficial.

Another preparation which can be used is an infant diarrhoea preparation KLN (Tx 21), available from chemists. 3–4 drops of KLN can be given via a dropper or on a teaspoon three times a day.

(Sulphadimidine 33%, Tx 7) diluted 1 : 1 with water to 16.5% strength can be given at a dose of 3 ml three times a day for a maximum of 5 days.

If the guinea pig has become anorexic a useful appetite stimulant is Vetrumex (Tx 13), a preparation which is formulated for cattle to replace their gut's natural bacterial flora. 0.25–0.5 of a teaspoonful can be mixed with a little water and rosehip syrup (source of vitamin C), and this dose can be given daily.

An alternative method of repopulating the affected guinea pig's gut with natural bacterial flora is to feed it fresh droppings from a healthy guinea pig.

Once a guinea pig has recovered, a normal diet can be reintroduced very slowly over the following 3–4 weeks, but it may take several more weeks for the guinea pig to regain its former condition.

Antibiotic-induced diarrhoea

The administration of certain antibiotics alters the gut flora in such a way that it allows the intestines to become colonized with *Clostridium* spp. This bacterial proliferation takes place mainly in the caecum. These bacteria produce enterotoxins and cause a fatal enteritis and diarrhoea. The most toxic drugs appear to be those with a narrow spectrum against Gram-positive organisms. Broad-spectrum antibiotics are a little safer, but none are totally free from the risk of inducing this condition. Topical antibiotic preparations will also induce enterotoxaemia if the guinea pig is allowed to lick at them (see Chapter 11 for a list of drugs).

Prevention: Where possible the use of antibiotics should be avoided. If they are necessary they are best given subcutaneously or intramuscularly as the oral route carries a lesser safety margin.

If antibiotics must be used they are best given with a probiotic, e.g. live natural yogurt or Avipro (Tx 11 or 12) to protect the gut flora.

During a course of antibiotics the uptake of essential vitamins in the gut is also likely to be upset, and administration of vitamin drops concurrently with the antibiotic and in the recovery period is recommended, e.g. Abidec drops (Tx 45).

Colic

This may occur as a sporadic symptom on its own or may accompany a more serious complaint such as gastroenteritis or an abdominal catastrophe, e.g. a torsion.

Clinical signs: The affected animal may appear bloated and will be very tender on abdominal palpation.

Treatment: Non-specific colics will respond well to a kaolin or kaolin and morphine preparation (Tx 22) given 3–4 times daily. Alternatively, the guinea pig can be given 1–3 ml of vegetable oil orally. If the colic is a symptom of a more serious condition, the prognosis is poorer and treatment must be aimed at the cause of the problem.

Intussusception

Clinical signs: This condition has been recorded in a guinea pig after a bout of diarrhoea. The initial scouring appeared to resolve after 5 days and then the guinea pig began to pass small amounts of blood mixed with firm motions. A day later it passed a 10 cm section of gut and the condition resolved completely.

Gastric torsion

This condition is occasionally diagnosed at post-mortem. It causes sudden death which may or may not be preceded by a period of intense abdominal discomfort.

Red droppings

Occasionally the droppings may be well formed but appear to have a dark red coating which may seem like blood. This can usually be related to the feeding of beetroot and should not be a matter for concern. Similarly the urine may also be stained red.

Anorexia

A guinea pig may stop eating for a great variety of reasons and this may be a symptom of many disease conditions. However, it is possible on occasion for an individual to develop a non-specific anorexia in the absence of any other clinical signs.

Treatment: Provided that no other reason for the anorexia can be determined, the affected guinea pig can sometimes be stimulated into regaining its appetite by feeding it a mixture of live natural yogurt (Tx 11) (or other probiotic, e.g. Vetrumex, Tx 13), vitamin C, ground faecal pellets from a healthy guinea pig and a little soaked dry food. Pureed baby food (vegetables or cereal) can also be included in this mixture. This mixture provides a boost to the normal gastrointestinal flora and is a useful appetite stimulant. An injection of anabolic steroid and multi-B vitamins can also be tried.

6 THE MUSCULOSKELETAL SYSTEM

The feet

The guinea pig has four toes on each foreleg and three toes on each hind leg. Each toe has an associated pad. Each forefoot has a main pad and a pronounced stopper pad. Each hind foot also has a main pad and a stopper pad which extends along the volar aspect of the metacarpus to the hock joint.

Overgrown toenails

The nails of some guinea pigs never need trimming, whilst others require frequent attention, particularly on the front feet where they can grow right round under and into the foot. By the very nature of the soft bedding on which they are kept, this problem is fairly common.

Treatment: Regular nail trimming to just below the quick, which is clearly visible if the nails are white. If the quick is accidentally cut the end can be cauterized with a styptic (e.g. potassium permanganate).

If the nail has actually grown into the foot the open wound should be cleansed with a saline solution (Tx 52) and Dermisol cream (Tx 23) or a wound powder applied topically.

Polydactyly

Clinical signs: The presence of an extra toe or toes, usually on the hind legs. It is sometimes a consequence of close inbreeding.

Treatment: As the extra toes are often only attached by a loose piece of skin, breeders may pinch them off between their forefinger and thumb soon after birth. Alternatively they can be removed with a pair of sharp scissors and any subsequent bleeding should be cauterized with potassium permanganate as with dew claw removal in very young puppies.

Bent leg

This condition is occasionally noticed at birth. The front leg is usually affected and this condition is attributed to the position of the foetus in the uterus, although it may be due to a muscle contracture. With careful massage and gentle manipulation the condition may resolve after the first few days of life.

Corns and pressure points

Clinical signs: Corns are a proliferation of horny material between the toes on the underside of the foot. They are most common on the forefeet.

Pressure points have a similar thickening on the point of the hocks and they commonly occur during pregnancy when the hind legs are carrying more weight than usual.

If the hygiene of the hutch floor is poor, corns will readily become infected and lead to the development of pododermatitis.

Treatment: Any extra horn can be carefully removed with a sharp pair of scissors and the area cleaned with dilute povidone–iodine solution (Tx 50). Both corns and pressure points can be softened with a petroleum jelly (Vaseline) or Dermisol cream (Tx 23) which can be rubbed into the affected area twice daily. The hutch floor should be kept clean and any abrasive bedding materials should be avoided.

Pododermatitis

Clinical signs: Swelling and ulceration of the foot pad. In severe cases this may progress to osteoarthritis and amyloidosis of the liver, spleen, kidneys and adrenal glands.

Treatment: The cause of this condition is usually bacterial in origin. The most commonly isolated bacterium is *Staphylococcus aureus*. Treatment of advanced infections where there is marked swelling of the foot is rarely successful. The foot should be cleaned with an antiseptic solution and a topical antibiotic/corticosteroid cream (Tx 26) applied to the affected area. Systemic or parenteral antibiotics (Tx 1–9) should also be administered. If possible, the foot should be lightly dressed to prevent any pieces of hay and shavings from aggravating the sore.

An alternative treatment which has been reported to be successful is the injection of antibiotics directly into the affected foot pad. A dose of 0.2 ml lincocin sterile solution (Pharmacia and Upjohn Ltd) equivalent to 20 mg lincomycin is injected daily for 5–7 days.

Comment: This condition is generally associated with rough flooring and poor hutch hygiene resulting in feet abrasions which become readily contaminated. By improving the floor surface and with regular hutch cleaning the incidence of this condition should be reduced. Subclinical vitamin C deficiency may also predispose the guinea pig to pododermatitis.

Occasionally similar symptoms are seen as a consequence of a fungal infection, and in these cases treatment with a suitable fungicide can be tried e.g. enilconazole (Tx 17). Alternatively the foot can be treated with cream containing the anti-fungal agents tolnaftate and nystatin (Tx 19, Tinaderm-M) twice daily.

Paralysis and reluctance to move

Trauma

Guinea pigs are very susceptible to spinal trauma if they are accidently dropped or fall from their hutch.

Clinical signs: These are of acute onset and usually related to the time of a fall. The guinea pig's hind legs may be totally paralysed and the normal nervous reflexes are usually absent. Urinary incontinence is often an accompanying feature. There may also be a palpable deviation or fracture in the spine and pain around this area. If necessary the diagnosis can be confirmed by radiography.

Treatment: If the damage is severe euthanasia is the kindest option.

Viral

Clinical signs: The affected animal may appear hunched over and unable to raise its head. Other symptoms include pyrexia, or weight loss with gradual muscular weakness and hind-leg paralysis.

Treatment: Unsuccessful.

Osteoporosis

This occurs if guinea pigs are over-supplemented with vitamin D, e.g. in the form of cod-liver oil. This leads to calcium resorption from bone and subsequent bone weakness. One of the first clinical signs is paralysis of the hind legs. If the guinea pig is receiving a balanced diet of dry and green food this supplementation is unnecessary. Sun-dried hay and exposure to sun-light will provide the guinea pig with adequate amounts of this vitamin.

Treatment: The dietary imbalance must be corrected and any vitamin D supplementation must be stopped. It may be helpful to withhold hay for the first few days and give the affected guinea pig extra calcium in the form of Collo-Cal D (Tx 46).

Comment: Vitamin D is often given to enhance the lustre of the coat, but it can be harmful if over-supplementation occurs. It is better to use a com-bination of polyunsaturated fatty acids, e.g. Vitapet or evening primrose oil, for this purpose.

The diet of the guinea pig must contain the correct ratio of calcium : phosphorus (see metastatic calcification) and no more than 1600 iu of vitamin D per kg.

Metastatic calcification

This condition is also the result of an alteration in the delicate balance of calcium, phosphorus and vitamin D. An imbalance of magnesium and potassium is also involved. However, as commercial diets are now better formulated it is an infrequent problem.

Clinical signs: Metastatic calcification is most often seen in males over a year old and these exhibit joint stiffness, poor weight gain and death.

Pathology: Calcium deposits in skeletal muscle and other organs, espe-cially the stomach, colon, lungs and aorta.

Comment: This condition can be minimized by feeding diets with a cal-cium : phosphorus ratio of 1.5 : 1 and no more vitamin D than 1600 iu/kg. In practice this can be achieved by a balanced diet of cavy pellets, green foods, carrots and beetroot.

If hyperphosphataemia does occur this leads to a compensatory fall in blood calcium. This hypocalcaemia stimulates the release of parathyroid hormone and calcium is resorbed from bone and deposited in skeletal muscle and many organs in the body, especially in the colon, stomach, aorta and lungs. Hyperphosphataemia occurs when guinea pigs are fed diets low in magnesium and potassium, and the condition can be minimized by feeding diets that contain at least 0.35% magnesium.

Rickets

This condition (which is also due to vitamin D deficiency) is extremely rare, as a balanced diet provides adequate calcium, phosphorus and vitamin D. Problems may only occur if the guinea pigs are kept in poor light, as sunlight is necessary to stimulate the production of vitamin D in the skin.

Muscular dystrophy

Clinical signs: The affected animal is stiff and reluctant to move. Some individuals may develop spontaneous hind-leg weakness and paralysis.

Pathology: Microscopic lesions include coagulative necrosis, inflammation and proliferation of the sarcolemmal nuclei in skeletal muscle.

Treatment: This condition is due to a vitamin E deficiency. The diet should contain 50 mg of vitamin E per kg. Wheatgerm oil is a useful source of vitamin E.

Scurvy

Clinical signs: Unsteady gait, painful locomotion, haemorrhage from gums, swollen costochondral junctions and poor weight gain or gradual wasting. Sub-clinical scurvy may present as excessive salivation or just a lowering of the guinea pig's resistance to the development of other conditions.

Pathology: Lesions include haemorrhages in the subcutis and in skeletal muscle. Also there may be haemorrhages around the joints (especially the stifle) and on all serosal surfaces. Microscopically there is a disarray of the cartilage columns and fibrosis in areas of active osteogenesis.

Treatment: An affected animal must be given 50–100 mg vitamin C per day, preferably as drops given orally, until the condition resolves.

Comment: The condition is due to a deficiency of vitamin C (ascorbic acid). An adult guinea pig requires 10–30 mg of vitamin C per day. Supplementation can be achieved by dissolving soluble vitamin C tablets

(Tx 47) in the drinking water (average water consumption is 8 ml per 100 g bodyweight) or by provision of adequate greenstuffs. Beetroot and carrots contain 3 mg per 25 g of vitamin C, and cabbage and spinach contain 17–20 mg per 25 g. Most proprietory guinea pig pellets contain adequate amounts of this vitamin provided that they have not been stored for longer than 3 months. Rabbit pellets, however, may contain little or no vitamin C.

Guinea pigs lack the enzymes necessary to convert L-gulonolactone to L-ascorbic acid and therefore require a dietary supplement of ascorbic acid. The normal requirement is 10 mg per kg bodyweight and this increases twofold during pregnancy.

There is no risk of over-supplementation with this vitamin as any excess is excreted through the kidneys.

Systemic disease

Infections with bacteria such as *Bordetella* and *Streptococcus* spp. will also produce a hunched-up posture and the affected individual will be disinclined to move.

Fractures

Limb fractures are usually sustained as a result of a fall as a consequence of the guinea pig being dropped. Rib fractures and subsequent chest injury are commonly seen in guinea pigs housed with rabbits. These fractures are usually the result of a kick from the rabbit's powerful hind legs.

Treatment: Limb fractures will respond well to external fixation, providing that they are adequately immobilized. External support is usually required for 3–4 weeks. Even if the limb is not returned to its full function the guinea pig will be able to cope adequately.

Femoral fractures can be repaired with an intramedullary pin. Callus formation following a fracture will occur after 7–10 days, and once the fracture is healed (confirmed by a radiograph) the pin can be removed.

Osteomyelitis

Clinical signs: Lameness and swelling of one or more joints.

Treatment: Broad-spectrum antibiotics (Tx 1–9).

Comment: The most common bacterial agents are *Staphylococcus aur-*

eus, *Streptococcus moniliformis, Pasturella multocida* and other streptococcal species. This condition may be a sequel to pododermatitis, as the likely route of infection is via an abrasion on the foot. Prevention must include improving the standard of hutch hygiene and removal of any abrasive flooring.

Osteoarthritis

The most commonly affected joint is the stifle. Clinical signs of lameness and weight loss can occur in guinea pigs of 9 months and older. There may be an increase in synovial fluid of the joint and the diagnosis can be confirmed by radiography. If the guinea pig is in pain, one drop of Metacam (Boehringer Ingelheim Ltd.) equivalent to 0.1 mg meloxicam can be given orally once daily.

Osteosarcoma

These are uncommon tumours, accounting for around 1% of all reported neoplastic lesions.

They are seen as a painful, bony swelling in guinea pigs over 1 year of age. The best treatment is amputation; if this is not possible then analgesia should be given (see Osteoarthritis).

7 THE HEAD AND NECK

THE EYE

Microphthalmia

Clinical signs: The eye is small or non-existent and the guinea pig is therefore blind. This condition is generally associated with all white-coated guinea pigs which are a result of either a Dalmatian × Dalmatian or a roan × roan mating. The offspring are known as 'microphthalmic whites'. Both these breeds should only be mated with self-colours, or self-coloured carriers.

Comment: The gene producing the roan coat colour is associated with a lethal gene which produces abnormalities of the eyes and occasionally accompanying disorders of the digestive tract.

Foreign bodies

Hay seeds commonly find their way into the eyes of guinea pigs. If undetected they may cause corneal ulceration and corneal oedema.

Clinical signs: Blepharospasm, epiphora and ocular discharge. Often unilateral conjunctivitis.

Treatment: A drop of local anaesthetic (Ophthaine) can be placed in the eye and it should then be possible to remove the seed with forceps, or with a piece of damp cotton wool. If there has been no corneal damage, antibiotic/steroid drops (Tx 29, Neobiotic HC) can be used for the following few days. If corneal ulceration is present, a topical antibiotic preparation should be used alone (e.g. cephalonium Tx 27). Application of all preparations should be made frequently (four times daily if possible).

69

Corneal ulceration

This is a common sequel to a foreign body in the eye, or it may be the result of damage to the cornea by a sharp piece of straw. Corneal damage is evident and corneal oedema is generally present. If healing has begun, blood vessels will be seen running towards the ulcer from the scleral margin.

Corneal oedema may be seen in one-day-old guinea pigs caused unintentionally by their mother whilst cleaning them. However, it can also be due to entropion (see below).

Treatment: Topical application of an antibiotic eye preparation twice daily, e.g. cephalonium (Tx 27) or chlortetracycline (Tx 28) eye preparations. If necessary, the eye can be bathed with a dilute saline solution (Tx 52). If the ulcer is not severe it will heal in 7–10 days (see also treatment of foreign bodies above).

Conjunctivitis

Clinical signs: The conjunctiva are reddened and there may be epiphora or an ocular discharge. It is seen as a symptom of upper respiratory disease, as an allergic response, or secondary to irritation and local trauma. In the last case the condition is usually unilateral, whilst bilateral conjunctivitis is usually a symptom of a more generalized condition.

A transient conjunctivitis associated with *Candida albicans* has also been recorded.

Treatment: If there is no corneal damage, topical applications of an antibiotic/steroid preparation (Tx 29) should be given three or four times daily.

If it appears to be a summer (pollen) allergy, a steroid eye preparation will be effective. A mild saline solution (Tx 52) applied to the eye by a dropper three times daily will also bring some relief to the affected individual. In allergy cases the swelling of the conjunctiva may also be accompanied by swelling of the eyelids.

Chlamydial neonatal conjunctivitis

Clinical signs: A bilateral conjunctivitis which is present at, or soon after, birth. There may be marked inflammation and chemosis.

Treatment: Use of an eye preparation containing chlortetracycline (Tx 28) three times daily.

Comment: Chlamydia can be associated with conjunctivitis in older animals. The incubation period may be as long as 6–8 weeks, and symptomless carriers do exist. *Chlamydia* is difficult to isolate from routine eye swabs, as it requires a special transport medium and specific test (PCR test). It may therefore be overlooked as a diagnosis of conjunctivitis in the older guinea pig, but should be considered if a stud suffers from an 'epidemic' of conjunctivitis. All affected and in-contact guinea pigs should be treated at the same time.

Entropion

Clinical signs: In-turning of the eyelid causing the eyelashes to rub against the cornea. This condition generally affects the lower eyelid and may be unilateral or bilateral. Affected youngsters will be born with corneal oedema or this may develop in the first few days of life. Minute areas of corneal ulceration may be visible.

Treatment: Often no treatment is required, although topical application of a suitable antibiotic eye preparation (Tx 27 or 28) will relieve the condition until the entropion corrects itself.

Comment: This condition is especially prevalent in the Texel breed. The corneal oedema will resolve after treatment and there is no permanent damage to the eye. The corneal damage occurs *in utero* whilst the eyes are shut, but since guinea pigs are born with their eyes open the eyelashes do not usually interfere with the cornea after birth. Most entropions which are present at birth correct themselves within the first 14 days of life.

Congenital cataracts

Cataracts which are present at birth have been seen in some lines of Abyssinians, and breeders may refer to this condition as 'mirror eye'. Related individuals may develop similar cataracts in early adulthood. The mode of inheritance is unknown, although studies suggest it may be sex-linked. None of the progeny from such an affected line should be used for further breeding.

Some youngsters may be born with partial cataracts which do not appear to progress as the guinea pig ages, and these small cataracts do not usually compromise vision.

Cataracts

Cases have been recorded where cataracts have developed when the guinea pig is 9–10 months old, and the condition is often unilateral. This is an inherited condition, although the mode of inheritance is unclear. It is advisable to remove the affected guinea pig and its progeny from the breeding programme as soon as the condition is diagnosed, otherwise it will reappear in future generations.

The author has also seen bilateral cataracts develop in a group of related guinea pigs at the age of 2–3 years. This condition also seems to be inherited and, as only sows are affected, it is therefore suggested that the mode of inheritance may be sex-linked. All types of inherited cataract are nuclear cataracts.

In cases of both unilateral or bilateral cataracts, the guinea pig is often able to cope adequately by relying on its senses of smell and hearing, especially if it is kept in familiar surroundings. In the early stages the pupillary light reflex is often still present, suggesting that the affected individuals may retain some degree of sight.

The development of cortical cataracts is associated with diabetes, or can be seen transiently during pregnancy.

Lens luxation

Bilateral lens luxation has been seen in an Abyssinian secondary to cataract formation.

On ophthalmic examination, an aphakic crescent is visible between the lens equator and the iris.

Adequate vision will be present unless the eye develops secondary glaucoma.

Milky ocular discharge

The presence of this discharge is often a cause for concern, but it is a normal fluid which is released from the eye as part of the grooming process. However, it must be differentiated from ocular discharges that accompany pathological changes in the eye.

'Fatty eye'

This is a term used to describe a permanent protrusion of the lower conjunctival sac. This condition is most common in Self-Whites, Blacks and

Creams and also Rexes. It is thought to be an inherited condition. The protrusion is caused by the presence of excess retrobulbar fat. If necessary the condition can be corrected by removing some of the fat through a small incision in the lower conjunctiva.

'Red eye'

This is a term used to describe a similar protrusion of the lower conjunctival sac. However, in contrast to 'fatty eye' this condition is not present all the time but appears at times of stress or when the eye is exposed to irritant substances such as cigarette smoke.

Treatment: A steroid eye preparation will reduce the inflammation.

THE EAR

Anatomy

The internal structure of the ear is essentially similar to that of all other mammals; however, the cochlea of the guinea pig has four coils, and they therefore possess very acute hearing. In comparison with the majority of other rodents the guinea pig has very large tympanic bullae.

Aural haematoma

Clinical signs: The pinna is swollen and feels full of fluid. It may be slightly warmer than normal. This condition must be differentiated from an abscess.

Treatment: This condition does not usually bother the affected guinea pig and it is probably best left alone to clot and shrink naturally by the process of clot resorption and fibrosis. However, if the guinea pig is a show animal an attempt can be made to drain the haematoma and reduce the swelling by suturing the ear between two buttons which will keep the pinna under constant pressure. The affected individual must be isolated, otherwise its companions are likely to chew at the sutures. The sutures should be left in for at least 2 weeks.

Wounds

These are usually a result of fighting. Tears and lacerations are common injuries which may be obtained during disputes over feeding bowls. Young guinea pigs may receive ear injuries if their mother is startled whilst she is feeding them and she accidentally catches their ears with her nails as she moves.

Treatment: If the wound is still bleeding, digital pressure should be applied. The ear should be held between finger and thumb for at least 5 minutes. If this is ineffective a small piece of Granuflex can be sutured over the wound. This will act as a pressure pad and also aid subsequent healing.

Older wounds can be bathed in a dilute salt solution (Tx 52) and dusted with an antiseptic wound powder.

Comment: Adequate numbers of feeding bowls must be provided to avoid head-to-head disputes over food.

Solar dermatitis

Clinical sign: This condition usually affects white guinea pigs with pink ears and occurs when they are exposed to sunlight. The pinnae become hot and inflamed.

Treatment: The affected guinea pig must be removed from the direct sunlight and the ears can be treated with a topical steroid cream (Tx 26).

Prevention: Affected guinea pigs should not be exposed to too much direct sunlight. Their ears can be protected by using an infant sunblocking preparation.

Middle ear disease

Clinical signs: The guinea pig holds its head over to the affected side and may fall over to the same side, due to a disturbance of its sense of balance.

Diagnosis: Pus may be seen in the ear canal. However, radiography of the tympanic bullae is often more useful than otoscopy as the changes in these large bullae are usually severe. Radiography will reveal a marked thickening of the bone of the tympanic bullae diagnostic of otitis media, and this may be present in the absence of a purulent discharge.

Treatment: This is generally unrewarding, as antibiotics, either parenteral or intra-aural, fail to reach the centre of the infection. If the guinea pig is otherwise well and is a single pet it is better left and allowed to compensate for its altered posture. Guinea pigs that are part of a large breeding unit are better destroyed to avoid the risk of the spread of infection.

Comment: This condition must be differentiated from wry neck, a congenital problem which causes a deformity in newborn guinea pigs, and which will also cause the guinea pig to hold its head over to one side (see p. 80). Middle ear disease may progress to affect the inner ear and subsequently the adjacent part of the meninges and brain. In these cases the clinical signs of circling, falling to the affected side and torticollis will persist.

This syndrome is often a sequel to a purulent upper respiratory tract infection associated commonly with *Streptococcus* and *Pasturella* spp. However, it may also accompany respiratory tract infections yet remain clinically inapparent. Otitis media is a common finding at post-mortem in individuals which have never exhibited clinical signs associated with this condition.

THE MOUTH

The teeth

Anatomy

The guinea pig has two upper and two lower incisors for gnawing. These teeth only have enamel on their front surfaces and are therefore self-sharpening. The canines are absent but in their place is a gap known as the diastema. There are four upper and lower cheek teeth (one premolar and three molars) on both sides. Guinea pigs' teeth are open-rooted and grow continuously (hypsodontic) and therefore they must be provided with a constant supply of hard food to ensure even wearing of the teeth.

Congenital absence of teeth: On rare occasions young are born without any teeth, and although they appear normal for the first 24 hours they then take on a starved hunched appearance as they cannot eat. They should be culled as they will not grow teeth later. As this is a genetic fault the parents of these affected young should not be bred from again.

Microphthalmic White guinea pigs are born with teeth abnormalities, malocclusion, or the absence of teeth. Such guinea pigs have eye and gut abnormalities concurrently and depending upon their disabilities do not survive for long.

Broken teeth

These commonly occur as a result of falls or fighting.

Treatment: The teeth must be clipped level to provide an even bite surface. It is doubly important that the guinea pig is supplied with hard foods at this time to keep the teeth even, as the feeding of soft foods will lead to uncontrolled growth of the other teeth.

Weak teeth

Clinical signs: The teeth break very easily, or may drop out if knocked.

Treatment: This can be a sign of vitamin D deficiency. Lack of this vitamin leads to a calcium deficiency and therefore poorly mineralized teeth and bones. The guinea pig acquires its vitamin D from two sources – from its diet and from the synthesis of vitamin D via its skin in daylight. It is only when it is deprived of both sources that teeth and bone weaknesses occur.

Excess vitamin D is harmful, but in severely affected cases one drop of cod-liver oil can be given orally for a week. At the same time the diet must be improved and the sunlight to the caviary increased. Alternatively a calcium and vitamin D supplement can be given (Tx 46).

Malocclusion

Molar malocclusion can be an inherited condition, or it can develop in any guinea pig over 1 year of age. The molar teeth wear unevenly, and the maxillary cheek teeth develop spurs which grow into and ulcerate the cheeks, whilst the mandibular cheek teeth grow towards the tongue causing buccal ulceration. In advanced cases the lower molars can grow across, and entrap the tongue.

Clinical signs: Salivation and weight loss. The guinea pig may still show interest in food, but be unable to masticate it.

Treatment: The guinea pig can be sedated so that the mouth can be examined. Special mouth gags and cheek pouch dilators are available for this purpose. The teeth can be trimmed and filed as necessary. Unfortunately some guinea pigs fail to improve after dental work. If the guinea pig has been anorexic for a while before presentation it is likely to have an associated fatty liver and ketosis which may be irreversible. Some guinea pigs develop a situation where they are unable to close their jaw properly to masticate, and this can occur unrelated to malocclusion.

Analgesia and vitamin C supplementation are essential after dental work, and the patient may need to be syringe fed initially to help maintain a positive energy balance. Because the teeth continue growing, dental work may be required every 6–8 weeks.

Comment: Similar symptoms are seen with 'wasting disease', a weight loss and salivation not associated with malocclusion. This condition can sometimes be attributed to vitamin C deficiency, or recently diabetes mellitus has been implicated as a cause. Vitamin C is a necessary precursor for collagen synthesis, and collagen is necessary to keep the teeth firmly fixed in their sockets. If the teeth loosen the guinea pig develops malocclusion.

Molar malocclusion is very common in Satins, yet is not seen in satin carriers. Teeth abnormalities are closely associated with the satin gene, which is a recessive gene.

Tooth root abscesses

Clinical signs: The guinea pig stops eating and may salivate profusely. Occasionally pus may be seen coming from the back of the mouth. The molars are usually affected by this condition and they can be examined satisfactorily by using an aural speculum (preferably metal).

Treatment: Broad-spectrum antibiotics (Tx 1–9) can be tried, but usually once the condition is detected the guinea pig is unlikely to respond and start eating again. A special mouth gag is required if the tooth is to be removed under general anaesthesia, as the anatomy of the mouth with the abundance of loose buccal skin does not lend itself easily to this kind of procedure.

Cleft palate

This congenital abnormality is obvious a few days after birth. The affected guinea pig is unable to suckle properly and food may be seen running down the nose. The cleft usually involves the hard palate only, and may vary from a small defect to the severe case which runs the whole length of the hard palate. There is no treatment for this and the guinea pig should be destroyed. As the condition is inherited the parents of the affected individual should not be bred from again.

Ptyalism (slobbers)

Slobbering can occur as a result of overgrown teeth, as a symptom of heatstroke, and it is also seen in cases of hypovitaminosis C. Salivation may also be a clinical sign of ketosis.

The lips

Scabs around the mouth: mild form

Clinical signs: The guinea pig has multiple scabs especially in the corners of the lips. If the condition is severe these can spread up over the nose. The affected animal is usually still in good health and eating normally.

Treatment: Cleanse the scabs around the mouth with an antiseptic solution daily. A dilute solution of povidone–iodine (Tx 50) is recommended. Panolog ointment or cream (Tx 25) should then be applied twice daily to the affected area. Alternatively the sores can be painted with gentian violet. The latter is the preferred method of treatment if the affected guinea pig is pregnant as antibiotics are best avoided during gestation.

Scabs around the mouth: severe form

Clinical signs: The scabs may progress to include the gums, and in turn the teeth may become brittle. Septicaemia and death are common.

Treatment: This condition is incurable and euthanasia should be considered.

Comment: Both forms are contagious and are spread via infected food dishes and drinkers and wire doors.

The milder form is more common. It is wise to isolate the affected guinea pig once the condition is diagnosed and the treatment should be successful, although there may be a recurrence of the condition at a later date.

The bacteria usually gain entry via small abrasions at the edges of the mouth from sharp pieces of food or from constant chewing by the guinea pig at its bars. It is wise to remove all abrasive foodstuffs to minimize the occurrence of this problem. All food bowls and drinkers should be sterilized, and the wire fronts of the hutch doors scrubbed with an antiseptic (e.g. dilute Savlon solution Tx 51).

The eating of foods with a high acid content may predispose the guinea pig to the development of this condition, and beetroot and apples should be removed from the affected individual's diet.

Recently a pox virus has been implicated as a cause of mouth scabs.

Sialitis

Clinical signs: Swelling of the throat in the region of the salivary glands and excess salivation.

Pathology: The formation of large eosinophilic intranuclear inclusion bodies in the epithelium of the salivary duct.

Comment: This may be due to a viral infection (cytomegalovirus). There is no treatment, but the condition may resolve with supportive therapy. Often the infection may be asymptomatic.

THE NECK

Cervical lymphadenitis

Clinical signs: Large, often unilateral swellings or abscesses in the ventral region of the neck. These swellings are in the cervical lymph nodes and are usually caused by an infection with *Streptococcus zooepidemicus*, although other bacteria can cause the same condition. In some cases death may occur as a result of septicaemia. Stress increases the guinea pig's susceptibility to infection.

Treatment: If possible, the lumps should be removed surgically. If this is not an option the abscesses should be lanced and flushed with chlorhexidine. Antibiotics should be given, either enrofloxacin or cephalexin (Tx 1 or 2). Recurrence is common as the treated animal may become a carrier.

Comment: Streptococcus zooepidemicus is normally present in the conjunctiva and nasal passages of guinea pigs. The causal organism usually gains access to the lymph nodes via abrasions of the oral mucosa or via the upper respiratory tract. Thus the use of abrasive materials in the feed or bedding should be avoided. As the material from discharging abscesses is highly contagious the affected animal should be isolated for treatment. If the animal is part of a large breeding colony it may be advisable to cull it to prevent the disease becoming enzootic.

Other bacteria which are frequently isolated are *Streptococcus moniliformis*, *Fusiformis* and *Pasteurella* spp.

Prevention: A clean, stress-free environment, and a good diet.

Foreign bodies

Clinical signs: A swelling in the throat region which is not associated with a lymph node. It may be hot and painful on palpation.

Comment: These abscesses are usually the result of a thistle from the hay which penetrates the mucous membranes of the mouth and tracks under the chin.

Treatment: If the abscess bursts, it can be bathed with a saline solution (Tx 52) and then flushed with 3% hydrogen peroxide (Tx 49). A topical preparation such as Dermisol (Tx 23) can then be used to assist healing.

If the abscess has not burst, it can be brought to a head by the use of warm poultices, and then treated as above.

If the position or size of the abscess is such that it compromises swallowing or causes great discomfort to the guinea pig it should be lanced and drained. It may be necessary to administer a general anaesthetic for this procedure.

Lymphosarcoma

Clinical signs: This may present as cervical lymphadenopathy. As the disease progresses there may be a more generalized lymphadenopathy, and hepatomegaly.

Diagnosis: Lymph node aspirate or biopsy.

Treatment: The condition has a poor prognosis. A high dose of prednisolone (2 mg/kg) can be given once daily.

Wry neck

This condition is seen in newborn guinea pigs. The severity of the condition is variable. The young exhibit degrees of torticollis, and those which are very badly affected may have to lie on their backs to suckle due to their abnormal head posture. More mildly affected individuals with only a slight deformity will be able to compensate and will appear near normal after 2–3 days.

This condition is hereditary and the parents of affected offspring should not be used for breeding again.

The thymus

In young guinea pigs this organ is present and palpable subcutaneously on either side of the trachea and within the neck. This is a clinically normal finding and should not be mistaken for a pathological condition.

8 BEHAVIOUR AND THE CENTRAL NERVOUS SYSTEM

Aggression

This is usually only a problem if boars are housed together. It is best to pen adult boars separately or with other females. Two young boars from the same litter may live in harmony if there are no females present. However, as they reach adulthood one will begin to exert its dominance and they may start fighting.

There is often an initial show of aggression when guinea pigs are penned together for the first time, but this will generally only be temporary, and will settle down once the 'pecking order' has been established. The aggressive animal will adopt a defensive posture and chatter its teeth in warning. The hair on its neck and shoulders may stand erect. These conflicts should not last longer than 2–3 hours, and if they do it is better to separate the offenders.

One procedure that can be tried to minimize this problem is to smear a little mentholated vapour rub (e.g. Vick) around the rump and under the chin of the original guinea pigs and of the newcomers. This eliminates the differences in the body odours of the two groups and often removes the trigger for conflict. It is also advisable to mix the two groups in mutual surroundings so that territory-protecting is not a component of any disagreements.

Unfortunately some sows may become aggressive when housed with other sows. Often the introduction of a boar will quieten an aggressive sow, or if necessary, she can be removed from the pen and housed separately with a boar.

It is important to provide plenty of food, and if necessary two or more bowls of dry mix in order to keep any disputes over feeding space to a minimum.

Epilepsy

Clinical signs: The affected guinea pig has a classic epileptic fit which can last for anything up to 3–4 minutes, during which time it salivates profusely and lies on its side twitching its limbs. There then follows a post-ictal period when it may exhibit abnormal behaviour such as polyphagia and aggression.

Treatment: Often, because the frequency of the fits increases, the affected animals are euthanased. The use of an anti-convulsant such as primidone (Tx 42, Mysoline) is a suggested alternative.

Fits

Guinea pigs may also have fits which are not true epileptiform convulsions. The fits may take the form of mild twitching or full seizures. They are usually secondary to another disease process and the prognosis is poor. Euthanasia is often the necessary outcome.

Fits such as these occur as a result of liver and kidney failure, ketosis, enterotoxaemia and septicaemia. They may also occur in guinea pigs with severe mycosis.

Convulsions may also be seen in guinea pigs which are very badly affected with severe pruritus caused by *Trixacarus caviae*, the mange mite. If the mange is treated successfully the fits will cease. Whilst ectoparasitic treatment is in progress any seizures can be controlled with diazepam (Tx 44) given by intramuscular injection at a dose of 1–2 mg/kg. Affected guinea pigs can then be maintained on primidone (Tx 42, Mysoline suspension).

Neonatal neurological deficits

Varying degrees of brain damage may be seen in youngsters which have suffered the trauma of a lengthy and difficult birth. These youngsters are often very uncoordinated and are unable to suckle properly. Hand-rearing is unsatisfactory as the affected young are unable to compensate for their disabilities, and euthanasia should be the considered option.

Foetuses which suffer central nervous defects of a genetic nature are usually aborted, or are stillborn.

Cerebellar disease

Clinical signs: Torticollis. The guinea pig may circle to one side, and may also fall over to the same side. Nystagmus seems to be a very infrequent clinical sign in affected guinea pigs.

Comment: These signs are almost always secondary to a middle ear infection which has progressed to the inner ear and the meninges. Encephalopathies leading to torticollis are very rare.

Similar symptoms have been seen following a cerebrovascular accident (CVA). Whatever the initiating cause of these symptoms the prognosis is poor.

Treatment: If a CVA is suspected, an injection of steroids (e.g. betamethasone, Tx 37) can be given. Treatment of middle ear disease with antibiotics is usually unrewarding, and if the guinea pig is part of a large breeding unit it is best to consider euthanasia as it is a potential source of infection for others.

9   HUSBANDRY

Introduction

There is a wealth of literature which is already available on this subject. The aims of this chapter are to discuss guinea pig management in relation to the prevention and treatment of disease conditions.

HOUSING

The commonest method of housing guinea pigs is in a hutch. However, they can be kept in a wide range of cage types, from converted cupboards to large cardboard boxes! Some guinea pigs are housed in wire cages with mesh floors.

Outdoor hutches can be covered with roofing felt, or a similar material, which will provide protection against bad weather. They should not be treated with creosote, as this is toxic to guinea pigs and will cause severe liver damage if the fumes are inhaled.

Size of accommodation

Each guinea pig should be allowed a minimum floor area of $0.2 \, \text{m}^2$. The cages should be at least 25 cm high.

However, a larger area for exercise is beneficial, and this can be provided either in the form of indoor floor runs, or as outdoor grass runs. The latter should be covered with mesh or netting to protect the guinea pigs from cats and other predators. The provision of adequate exercise is especially important for sows during pregnancy as it may help prevent the development of pregnancy toxaemia.

The flooring

If wire floors are used, care must be taken to ensure that there are no abrasive surfaces which could cause foot damage and subsequent podo-dermatitis. A mesh of 0.5 cm × 1 cm or smaller will prevent the guinea pigs trapping their feet in the wire holes.

The preferred bedding material is a layer of newspaper which is covered with woodshavings and hay. If woodshavings are used it is important that they are made only from untreated softwoods, as certain hardwoods have toxic properties. Sawdust is not recommended for use as a bedding material as it is too fine and particles may easily become lodged in the guinea pig's eyes if it tries to burrow under the bedding. Sawdust has also been found lodged in the prepuce of males, causing impaction and infection.

Straw is also not recommended as it is abrasive by nature, and is responsible for causing a large proportion of eye injuries.

Hygiene

The accommodation should be cleaned out regularly. If the litter is allowed to build up there will be an accumulation of ammonia and this weakens the resistance of the respiratory tract to infection.

As the guinea pig's urine often contains small crystals of ammonium phosphate and calcium carbonate there may be a build up of scale around the hutch. This can be removed by cleaning with a weak acid solution (e.g. dilute acetic acid).

Environment

The guinea pigs should be kept away from draughts and protected against extremes of temperature. They should receive adequate amounts of light, but should not be exposed to direct sunlight during the summer as they are very susceptible to the development of heatstroke (see below). Recom-mendations for the environmental temperature and humidity are:

- Temperature: 20–22°C (68–72°F)
- Humidity: 45–65%

These figures apply for optimum performance; however, guinea pigs can be quite safely kept at much lower temperatures (such as those we experience during our British winters) provided that they are protected from draughts. At temperatures above 29°C there is a high incidence of infertility problems and early abortions.

Heatstroke

Guinea pigs are prone to developing heatstroke when exposed to high environmental temperatures (above 28°C) or when kept in grass runs exposed to strong sunlight. Heavily pregnant females are the most susceptible, and the problem is worse if they are deprived of water at the same time. They are also particularly susceptible during car journeys to shows, and at shows too, if their show pen is in direct sunlight.

Clinical sign: Rapid respiration, salivation, prostration and eventually death.

Treatment: They must be cooled rapidly. If necessary their body can be immersed in cold water. An injection of steroids (e.g. betamethasone Tx 37) may be beneficial.

NUTRITION

Many disease conditions in guinea pigs can be related to the feeding of an incorrect diet. It is very important to provide a well-balanced diet and the following sections aim to discuss a few basic principles of guinea pig nutrition and describe the qualities of common foodstuffs and their relationship to disease conditions.

Principles of guinea pig nutrition

(1) The guinea pig, like humans and apes, is unable to synthesize its own vitamin C (ascorbic acid) as it lacks the enzyme L-gulonolactone oxidase which is required to convert L-gulonolactone to L-ascorbic acid. It therefore requires a daily supply of vitamin C. The normal requirement for vitamin C is 10 mg/kg, and this increases to 20 mg/kg during pregnancy.

　　If vitamin C is added to the drinking water in the form of soluble tablets (Tx 47) it must be given via a dish or a bottle with a stainless steel nozzle. Other metals will accelerate the decomposition of ascorbic acid. Rosehip syrup is a useful alternative which can be added to the drinking water to provide extra vitamin C. It should be diluted with water to produce a solution containing 12 mg of vitamin C per 100 ml.

The daily requirements for this vitamin will be met as long as a balanced diet of dry food, carrots and greens is fed. The vitamin C content of dried food will deteriorate over 9–12 weeks, so deficiency problems will arise if the dry food is stale. Rabbit food is also unsuitable as it does not contain adequate amounts of this vitamin.

Hypervitaminosis C is not a recognized problem as any ascorbic acid which is excess to requirements is excreted through the kidneys.

(2)   Any dietary change must be made slowly, e.g. the introduction of grass and hedgerow plants once their supply becomes plentiful in the spring. Sudden changes will cause diarrhoea and digestive disturbances.

(3)   A balanced diet must include the following every day:
 • Concentrates – the dry food
 • Roots – carrots or beetroot
 • Green foods – cultivated or hedgerow plants
 • Hay – of good quality
 • Fresh water
If this balance of diet is adhered to there should be little need for extra supplementation, except in a few special cases. Over-zealous vitamin and mineral supplementation may actually unbalance the diet and cause disease problems, e.g. vitamin D overdose if cod-liver oil is added to the diet.

Most of the required vitamins are actually synthesized by the intestinal flora.

(4)   All food should be fed fresh with no mould on it. Any dry food and greenstuffs which have not been eaten after a few hours should be removed and not allowed to rot in the hutch, as this will lead to digestive upsets.

(5)   Frosted food must not be fed as it will cause digestive upsets. Food should be allowed to thaw if it is kept in the refrigerator, and any fresh food remaining in the hutch should be removed at night during the cold winters as it is likely to freeze overnight.

(6)   The diet of a young guinea pig should be as varied as possible. It is at this age that the guinea pig is learning about foodstuffs and what it will

eat as an adult reflects what it was fed as a youngster. If a guinea pig is offered a new food as an adult it is unlikely to accept it unless it starts to copy other adults in the pen which may be eating it.

(7) As the guinea pig is always eating, a supply of hay must be constantly available to prevent boredom. Guinea pigs which have plenty of hay to eat are less likely to develop vices like hair chewing.

Deficiency diseases

Scurvy

This is the result of a vitamin C deficiency. Sub-clinical deficiency lowers the guinea pig's resistance and predisposes it to the development of bacterial pneumonia, acute enteritis and skin conditions, especially ringworm.

Clinical sign: General unthriftiness, poor weight gain and gradual wasting. Also reluctance to move and lameness. Less commonly seen are haemorrhages from the gums. Excess salivation may be seen in sub-clinical cases.

Pathology: Haemorrhages in the subcutis and in skeletal muscle. Haemorrhages around the joints, especially the stifle, and on all serosal surfaces. Microscopically there is disarray of the cartilage columns and fibrosis in areas of active osteogenesis.

Treatment: Affected cases should be given 50–100 mg/kg vitamin C a day, preferably as drops, until the condition resolves.

Comment: See notes on vitamin C at the beginning of the nutrition section.

Muscular dystrophy

This is due to an alpha-tocopherol (vitamin E) deficiency. Guinea pigs are particularly sensitive to this deficiency. However, if the guinea pig is receiving a properly balanced commercial diet this deficiency is unlikely to arise.

Clinical signs: Stiffness and reluctance to move. Some guinea pigs show spontaneous hind-leg weakness and paralysis.

Pathology: A coagulative necrosis, and inflammation and proliferation of the sarcolemmal nuclei in skeletal muscle.

Treatment: Adequate provision of vitamin E. The diet should contain 50 mg/kg of feed. Affected individuals can be given wheatgerm oil as a liquid form of vitamin E. Vitamin E tablets can be given at a dose of 5–10 mg/kg daily.

Comment: A diet lacking in vitamin E may also lead to infertility problems.

Metastatic calcification

This condition is secondary to an alteration in the complex relationship between calcium, phosphorus, magnesium and potassium. However, as commercial diets are now better formulated, this is an infrequent problem.

Clinical signs: This condition is seen most commonly in boars over 1 year of age. Soft tissue deposits of calcium may lead to lameness, joint stiffness, unthriftiness and death, or they may just be an incidental finding at post-mortem examination.

Pathology: Calcium deposits are found in the colon, stomach, aorta and lungs. Many other organs may also be affected.

Comment: This condition can be minimized by feeding diets with a calcium : potassium ratio of 1.5 : 1 and no more vitamin D than 1600 iu/kg. In practice this can be achieved by feeding a balanced diet of good hay, dry food, greens, carrots and beetroot.

Atrophy or 'wasting disease'

Clinical signs: This condition is characterized by weight loss, especially of the hind legs and flanks, which may progress to paralysis, a scurfy coat and salivation. The affected guinea pig continues to eat well despite the progression of the disease.

Comment: The aetiology of this condition is unclear. It is often considered to be due to a vitamin deficiency, particularly of vitamin C. Overgrown teeth have also been implicated as the cause. However, some affected guinea pigs have no teeth problems and are fed a balanced diet. Recently diabetes mellitus has been suggested as a possible cause.

Treatment: The molars can be checked using an aural speculum, and if they are overgrown they can be clipped. However, the problem is likely to recur as they will continue to grow (see Chapter 7).

If the diet is inadequate it must be improved. Vitamin C can be given at 100 mg per day until the condition resolves.

One reported case resolved with a good diet and intensive nursing which included daily warm baths and hind-leg massage.

Unfortunately not all cases recover, and in the case of severely affected guinea pigs euthanasia should be considered.

Vitamin K deficiency

Clinical signs: Epistaxis, intra-uterine haemorrhage, post-partum haemorrhage seen especially in guinea pigs fed only on poor hay and stale dry food.

Treatment: An injection of vitamin K can be given intramuscularly (Konakion, Roche) at a dose of 0.5–1 mg/kg. Vitamin K can then be given orally, and the diet should be improved.

Comment: The recommended requirement of this vitamin is 2 mg/kg of feed.

Food values of cultivated crops

Beetroot: Contains folic acid, calcium, iron, sodium and vitamin C (3 mg per 28 g), also vitamins B_1 and B_2. Too many leafy tops must not be fed as they contain high levels of oxalic acid which will cause acute renal failure.

Broccoli: Contains vitamins A and B_2, folic acid and vitamin C (17–20 mg per 28 g). Both white and purple sprouting varieties can be fed.

Brussel sprouts: The leaves of these plants can be given. They contain vitamin C (17–20 mg per 28 g) and also vitamins A and B_6, and folic acid.

Cabbage: Contains vitamins A and B_6, folic acid and vitamin C (17–20 mg per 28 g). It also contains calcium, iron, copper and potassium. Guinea pigs will eat green and spring cabbage, but will not always touch the harder white cabbage.

Carrot: Contains calcium, iron, sodium and vitamins A, B_1, B_2, B_6 and C (3 mg per 28 g). The carrot tops are also enjoyed.

Celery: Contains 2 mg of vitamin C per 28 g, and also vitamins A and B_1. The leaves and stalks can both be fed.

Cauliflower: The outside leaves can be given and their food value is approximately the same as cabbage.

Lettuce: Should only be fed in small amounts. It contains 3 mg of vitamin C per 28 g, but it also contains the substance laudanum, which can be harmful.

Spinach: This contains calcium, iron, sodium, potassium and magnesium. It also contains vitamins A, B_2, B_6, E and C, and folic acid (17–20 mg/kg).

Swede: This contains 7 mg of vitamin C per 28 g, but its quality rapidly deteriorates in storage and it readily goes dry and fibrous.

Watercress: This can be fed as a treat. It contains calcium and sodium and vitamins A and C, and folic acid.

Food values of fruit

Apple: Contains 1 mg of vitamin C per 28 g. Apples can be fed as a treat, but not given in large quantities as they are fairly acidic.

Wild plants

Plants collected from the hedgerows provide a varied and interesting diet. They must be:

- Collected away from areas soiled by dogs
- Free from bird droppings
- Not from areas where weedkiller or pesticide has been used
- Not from roadsides close to car exhaust fumes

See Table 9.1 for a list of poisonous plants which must be avoided.

The main principle of feeding hedgerow plants is to provide the guinea pig with a balance of plants with laxative and those with astringent properties. If too many with a laxative effect are fed diarrhoea will occur, and conversely excess astringents may lead to constipation. However, these properties can be used beneficially to correct digestive disturbances and the feeding of astringents only may resolve a case of diarrhoea of dietary origin.

Table 9.1 Poisonous plants. These include *all* plants that grow from bulbs

Bracken	Horsetails
Bryony	Lily of the valley
Buttercup (this is safe if fed dried in hay)	Mayweeds
Charlock	Monkshood
Convolvulus (bindweed)	Privet
Deadly nightshade	Ragwort
Foxglove	Speedwell
Hellebore	Toadflax
Hemlock	Wild celery
Henbane	

Astringents

- Bramble leaves (with the thorns removed)
- Shepherd's purse (see Fig. 9.1)
- Docks. These must only be fed before the flower stalks appear. After this their content of oxalic acid rises and too many will cause renal failure
- Cleavers (goosegrass) (see Fig. 9.2)

Fig. 9.1 Shepherd's purse.

Fig. 9.2   Cleavers (goosegrass).

Laxatives

- Dandelions
- Groundsel (see Fig. 9.3)

Other plants

- Grass is a very valuable food during the summer and the guinea pig can live in a grass run all day. Care must be taken if feeding grass clippings as they overheat very quickly and cause diarrhoea
- Sow thistle. Useful for lactating sows
- Vetches
- Yarrow (see Fig. 9.4)
- Coltsfoot. This was used as an old remedy for treating colds and asthma

Dry food

In this category are pellets and cereals (bran, oats, barley and flaked maize). The pellets should contain adequate quantities of vitamin C, although this will deteriorate if they are stored for over 6 weeks. Excess rabbit pellets may cause 'broken back' (see Chapter 1). This condition may also occur if too much flaked maize or barley is included in the diet as both of these foods have overheating properties.

As all foodstuffs in this category are of high calorific value they must not be fed in large quantities to pregnant sows as an obese sow is more prone

Fig. 9.3 Groundsel.

to developing pregnancy toxaemia or dystocia. The practice of feeding molasses-enriched mixes must be considered carefully because these too are high in calories.

The nutritional requirements of the guinea pig are as follows:

(1) For maintenance
  - Oil: 2.6%
  - Protein: 13%
  - Fibre: 8%
  - Ash: 6.5%

(2) For breeding
  - Oil: 3.5%
  - Protein: 18%
  - Fibre: 11.2%
  - Ash: 7.3%

Fig. 9.4 Yarrow.

Some dry mixes sold for small animals in pet shops do approximate quite closely to these requirements. The protein content is the most important factor as diets too low in protein will lead to retarded growth and reduced breeding capacity, whereas diets too high in protein (over 22%) may lead to an increased incidence of abortions.

If a suitable petfood mix is unavailable, some goat mixes and riding pony mixes will make suitable alternatives.

A simple means of giving a mixture of cereals is to give them in a bran mash, although some guinea pigs may not eat it in this form. Bran can be fed soaked in water mixed with breadcrumbs or as a soaked mix of oat-meal, wheatmeal and bran in the ratio $1:2:3$.

This can be fed daily in winter and less frequently during the summer and throughout pregnancy. In times of increased vitamin requirement (e.g. during the winter) a vitamin syrup such as Minadex can be added to the mash. As bran is low in calcium and high in phosphorus, too much during pregnancy may lead to the development of young with a poorly mineralized bone structure.

Rabbit food contains too little vitamin C and also excess vitamin D (which may lead to metastatic calcification). Some rabbit pellets for commercial rabbit production contain coccidiostats; these are unnecessary drugs for guinea pigs and have been associated with stunted growth and sporadic deaths when inadvertently fed to guinea pigs. The majority of coccidiostats are ionophores and these have a harmful effect on the natural flora of the gut, and although they may not induce diarrhoea they decrease the digestive efficiency of the guinea pig's gut and this leads to sub-optimal growth rates in the affected stock. If rabbits are kept with guinea pigs, it is better to feed them both a proprietary guinea pig mix which will be suitable for both.

Aflatoxicosis

This is an infrequent condition, but it may be seen if dry food (especially maize) is stored in damp warm conditions and becomes contaminated with *Aspergillus flavus*.

Clinical signs: Varying degrees of hepatotoxicity, depending upon the amount of contaminated food consumed. Mildly affected cases will become lethargic and inappetent, whilst more acute cases will exhibit loss of coordination, convulsions and death.

Pathology: An exudative hepatitis in acute cases. Chronic cases will have cirrhotic livers.

Treatment: None.

10 ANAESTHETICS AND SURGICAL PREPARATIONS

Guinea pigs do not make particularly good anaesthetic candidates as their response to anaesthesia is extremely variable, especially if an injectable agent is used. It is always best to use a familiar anaesthetic when contemplating any form of surgery on a guinea pig; however, there are many different methods of anaesthetizing this species which have been documented in the literature and this chapter will discuss them all. Other important considerations which will contribute to the success of any procedure are careful preparation for surgery and intensive post-operative nursing.

Preparation for surgery

Before anaesthesia the guinea pig should, where possible, be fasted for at least 2 hours to make its response to the anaesthetic more predictable and to ensure its mouth is clear of food (guinea pigs are unable to vomit).

If an inhalation agent is used, atropine is a useful premedicant as it will reduce salivation during the anaesthetic period. A dose of 60 µg/kg should be administered by subcutaneous injection.

One of the major problems of anaesthesia in any small animal is that of heat loss during surgery, and there are several ways that this heat loss can be minimized:

(1) The patient can be placed on a heat-reflective surface, e.g. 'Flectabed'.

(2) The patient can be wrapped in aluminium foil with only the operation site exposed.

(3) Extra heat can be provided by using a heat lamp above the operating table.

The patient should not be placed on a hot water bottle as this will encourage vasodilation, and therefore increase heat loss.

The operation site should be clipped and then cleaned with a suitable anti-bacterial solution, e.g. povidone–iodine (Tx 50) and then sprayed with surgical spirit. Do not overwet the patient as this will cause further heat loss due to the evaporation of these fluids. The cleaning solution should be used at body temperature.

The time taken for the preparation and the surgery itself should be kept to a minimum in order to cause as little stress to the patient as possible.

Depth of anaesthesia

This can be monitored by pinching either the ears or the webs of the toes. Once the responses to these stimuli disappear surgical anaesthesia has been achieved.

INHALATION ANAESTHETICS

Induction

This is best carried out by placing a small facemask over the guinea pig's head, and supporting the guinea pig on the table by placing cupped hands over its body. During induction guinea pigs exhibit a normal squirming activity. This does not mean that they are fighting the anaesthetic and the induction concentration must not be raised as this will increase the risk of overdosage. There is a greater risk of overdosing with halothane than with methoxyflurane during induction.

Circuit

It is best to use an Ayre's T piece and a small facemask both for induction and maintenance. If a small enough facemask is unavailable one can easily be constructed from a plastic syringe case.

Halothane

This is the most commonly used anaesthetic in veterinary surgeries and it can safely be used as an anaesthetic in this species.

Induction can be achieved using a 3% concentration, with the anaesthesia maintained with a lower concentration of between 1 and 2%. This can either be used with oxygen alone or a 1 : 1 mixture of nitrous oxide and oxygen.

Isoflurane

If this is available this is the most suitable inhalation anaesthetic for guinea pigs. Induction can be achieved with a 3% concentration and maintenance with a 1–2% concentration with oxygen. As the anaesthetic is 98% eliminated by the lungs there is no 'hangover' period after anaesthetic administration.

INJECTABLE ANAESTHETICS

All injections should be made into the quadriceps using a 23–26 gauge needle. Where possible no more than 0.3 ml should be injected at any one site, and thus in some cases the anaesthetic dose must be divided and injected equally into different muscle masses.

Hypnorm

Hypnorm (Janssen Animal Health) contains fentanyl (a morphine analgesic) and fluanisone (a neuroleptic) and it can be used to provide either sedation and light anaesthesia, or deeper anaesthesia if used in combination with diazepam (Valium, Roche).

Dose: 1 mg/kg given intramuscularly for sedation. 1 mg/kg given intramuscularly plus 2.5 mg/kg of diazepam given as an intraperitoneal injection for surgical anaesthesia. Naloxone (Narcan) given at a dose rate of 0.1 mg/kg given intraperitoneally or intramuscularly will reverse the anaesthesia.

Comment: The use of fentanyl has been associated with the development of tissue necrosis at the injection site, and also self-mutilation of the distal limb in which the injection was given.

Ketamine

Vetalar (Pharmacia and Upjohn Ltd.) contains 100 mg/ml of ketamine.

Dose: 100 mg/kg given intramuscularly will provide good immobilization but little analgesia. It is a useful form of restraint for minor procedures.

Comment: The administration of ketamine has been associated with self-mutilation of the distal limb in which the injection was given.

Ketamine and xylazine

Ketamine can also be used in conjunction with xylazine (Rompun, Bayer) to produce deep anaesthesia. The two drugs can be mixed together and are then best given in a divided dose intramuscularly.

Dose: Ketamine 60 mg/kg and xylazine 8 mg/kg will produce anaesthesia in 15–20 minutes. Ketamine 100 mg/kg and xylazine 4 mg/kg will produce anaesthesia in 12–15 minutes. The guinea pig should be kept in a darkened and quiet place until anaesthesia develops. The sedation can be reversed with atipamezole (Antisedan, Pfizer Ltd.) at a dose of 1 mg/kg subcutaneously.

Ketamine and medetomidine

Ketamine can be combined with medetomidine to produce sedation adequate for dental work.

Dose: Ketamine (40 mg/kg intramuscularly) and medetomidine (Domitor Pfizer Ltd.) at a dose of 0.5 mg/kg intramuscularly. The sedation can be reversed using atipamezole (Antisedan, Pfizer Ltd.) at a dose of 1 mg/kg subcutaneously.

Post-anaesthetic complications

These include respiratory infections, digestive disturbances, generalized depression and inappetance. However, many of these problems can be overcome with good nursing and post-operative care.

Immediate post-operative care

If respiration is depressed during or after surgery, doxapram hydrochloride (Tx 39) should be given at a dose of 10–15 mg/kg either subcutaneously or intramuscularly.

After surgery the patient should be kept in a warm box and allowed to recover. The optimum temperature of the recovery area should be 25–30°C (75–85°F).

15 ml of fluids (Tx 15, glucose–saline) can be administered subcutaneously. These should be gently warmed before their administration.

Analgesia

Guinea pigs should receive analgesia following surgery; this will significantly improve their recovery rate.

Buprenorphine can be given at a dose of 0.05 mg/kg by subcutaneous injection. Vetergesic (Animalcare Ltd.) contains 0.3 mg/ml buprenorphine, and this approximates to a dose of 0.17 ml/kg.

Butorphanol can be given at a dose of 2 mg/kg by subcutaneous injection. Torbugesic (Fort Dodge Animal Health) contains 10 mg/ml of butorphanol and this approximates to a dose of 0.2 ml/kg.

The convalescent patient

If the guinea pig's appetite is depressed following surgery further administration of subcutaneous fluids may be required. Alternatively, fluids can be given orally via a dropper or syringe. If anorexia continues for several days after surgery, the guinea pig must be given glucose in its oral fluid mixture to prevent the onset of ketosis. Oral vitamin C (20–30 mg/kg) should also be administered daily to the dehabilitated patient. Until the guinea pig begins to eat on its own it can be syringe fed with proprietary human convalescent food (e.g. Complan) or baby foods. Vetrumex (Tx 13) may also act as an effective appetite stimulant if given orally.

The patient must be constantly stimulated and encouraged. If left alone a sick guinea pig will give up quickly, but intensive nursing is often quite rewarding. The presence of another guinea pig will also provide some encouragement to the convalescent guinea pig and will often stimulate it to start feeding again.

The convalescent guinea pig must be kept in warm surroundings at a constant temperature. For the individual, a box in an airing cupboard will provide the perfect environment for the recovering guinea pig. Alternatively an external heat source should be provided, either in the form of a heat lamp or a domestic light bulb. Direct contact with a hot water bottle is not recommended as there is the risk of causing burns to the guinea pig, as well as stimulating vasodilation which would be deleterious to the shocked patient. However, if the guinea pig is placed in a box with an open mesh or grid above it, a hot water-bottle can be used as an overhead heat source if placed on this 'roof' and covered with a towel.

11 TREATMENTS

This chapter aims to summarize all the treatments mentioned in the preceding chapters and describe their modes of administration and dosage. Each drug is coded with a treatment (Tx) number for easy cross reference.

All the doses are given in milligrams (mg) or millilitres (ml) per kg. As a rough guideline an adult guinea pig weighs 1 kg, although some of the larger types may weigh up to 1400 g. The birth weight is between 75 and 100 g and their weight gain is approximately 4 g per day until they reach their adult weight at 8 months of age.

Routes of drug administration

Subcutaneous injection: This can be given under the skin at the scruff of the neck or, for larger volumes of injection, under the skin overlying the thorax. Up to 10 ml can be administered in this way. A 23–26 gauge needle should be used.

Intramuscular injection: This can be administered into the quadriceps muscles using a 23–26 gauge needle. The maximum volume given at one site is 0.3 ml. If a series of daily injections is to be given alternate hind legs should be used on subsequent days.

Intraperitoneal injection: The guinea pig is best held supported under its forelegs and bottom, and positioned on its back with its head held slightly lower than its hindquarters to allow the stomach and intestines to fall forward. The needle should be inserted to the right of the midline 2.5 cm in front of the pubis, and directed forwards at an angle of 45°. Up to 15 ml can be administered using a 23–25 gauge needle.

Intravenous injection: The veins of a guinea pig are very small and dosing via this route is difficult. The largest and most accessible veins are the ear veins and the bracheocephalic vein.

Oral dosing: This is the most frequently used route for drug administration in general practice as it is usually the most practicable. However, it is often associated with antibiotic toxicity as antibiotics given orally have a direct and undesirable effect on the natural gut flora (see later). It is very important to use oral antibiosis with great caution and only when it is really necessary.

Drops of liquid can be placed on the tongue via a dropper or a syringe. One drop from a 2 ml syringe is equivalent to 0.02 ml.

It is not generally recommended to mix antibiotics in the drinking water as the water intake of a sick guinea pig may be markedly reduced, whilst healthy individuals in the same pen may take in large and often toxic amounts of the antibiotic. An exception to this is if a colony problem is being treated (e.g. *Coccidium*).

Stomach tube: A pliable rubber or plastic tube with a diameter of 1.5–6 mm is recommended. The disadvantage of this method is that the guinea pig may need to be anaesthetized for this procedure and this is undesirable for most weak or debilitated patients.

Antibiotics

Antibiotics must be administered with caution as the guinea pig is very sensitive to the toxic effects of many of the commonly used antibiotics. This toxicity occurs because the antibiotics destroy the natural gut bacteria which enables the overgrowth of *Clostridia* spp., especially *Clostridium difficile*, as well as other Gram-negative species. This overgrowth causes a fatal enterotoxaemia leading to diarrhoea and death between 3 and 7 days after the administration of the antibiotic.

Antibiotics with a narrow spectrum of activity appear to be the most toxic, especially if the activity is against Gram-positive organisms. Antibiotics that have known toxic activity are:

- Ampicillin
- Bacitracin
- Erythromycin
- Lincocin
- Penicillin
- Streptomycin

- Tylosin
- Tetracycline (but see note, p. 108)

The risk of inducing enterotoxaemia is highest when using oral preparations as they have a direct effect on the bacterial flora of the gut. The incidence of side-effects is lower with parenterally administered antibiotics. Care must also be taken if using topical preparations as they can produce the same syndrome if licked by the affected guinea pig or its inmates.

The risk of toxicity can be reduced if the antibiotic is given concurrently with a probiotic (see later).

The simultaneous administration of a vitamin B complex may also help prevent these undesirable side-effects.

Before treating any individual with antibiotics one must be certain that the benefits outweigh the potentially harmful consequences.

ANTIBIOTICS

Tx 1. Enrofloxacin

Baytril (Bayer plc)

This broad spectrum bactericidal antibiotic is now the drug of choice for most infections.

Dose: 5–10 mg/kg daily. The 2.5% injection can be given the subcutaneous route at a dose of 0.3 ml/kg daily. The 2.5% oral solution can be diluted 1 : 1 with blackcurrant syrup (e.g. Ribena) to increase its palatability and this mixture given orally at a dose of 0.4 ml twice a day to an adult.

Tx 2. Cephalexin

Ceporex (Schering-Plough Animal Health)

This contains 180 mg/ml cephalexin.

Dose: 50 mg/kg by intramuscular injection daily. This approximates to a dose of 0.25 ml/kg.

The recommended dose should be given for 14 days when treating *Streptococcus zooepidemicus*.

Tx 3. Chloramphenicol

Chloramphenicol injectable suspension (Fort Dodge Animal Health)

This contains 150 mg/ml of chloramphenicol.

Dose: 20 mg/kg injected intramuscularly daily. This approximates to a dose of 0.15 ml/kg.

Chloramphenicol is the drug of choice for treating cases with central nervous system involvement as it readily crosses the blood–brain barrier.

Tx 4. Metronidazole

Torgyl (Merial Animal Health Ltd.)

This contains 5 mg/ml metronidazole.

Dose: 20 mg/kg once daily. This is equivalent to 4 ml/kg. It can be given orally, mixed with food or water, or injected subcutaneously. The major disadvantage of this is the large quantity of drug that must be injected, but the dose can be split and administered at two different sites, which will also lead to a faster rate of its absorption.

Tx 5. Neomycin

Neobiotic pump (Pharmacia and Upjohn Ltd.)

This contains 50 mg/ml of neomycin and 0.25 mg/ml of methscopolamine bromide. The latter is an anti-cholinesterase and helps combat bacterial enteritis.

Dose: The dose per guinea pig is 5 mg/kg twice daily. The drops are diluted 1 part drops : 4 parts water to produce a solution containing 10 mg/ml of neomycin, and the dose is 0.5 ml/kg twice daily. This should be given orally.

Neomycin is poorly absorbed from the digestive tract, and if it is used to treat infections elsewhere in the body it may fail to reach therapeutic levels at its required site of action.

Tx 6. Nitrofuratoin

This is a human drug which can be used in cases of cystitis. Furadantin 50 mg (Norwich Eaton) contains 50 mg of nitrofuratoin.

Dose: One tablet (50 mg/kg) a day for 3 days.

Tx 7. Sulphadimidine

Intradine (Norbrook Laboratories Ltd.)

This contains 0.33 g/ml sulphadimidine sodium.

Dose: The solution can be diluted 1 : 1 with water and 3 ml/kg given three times daily by oral administration. This is equivalent to a dose of 0.5 g/kg of sulphadimidine sodium three times daily.

   The treatment should not be continued for longer than 5 days.

   Alternatively, the drinking water can be replaced by a 0.2% solution of sulphadimidine sodium (1 ml of Intradine : 150 ml water).

   This sulphonamide can be given against the majority of infections and is particularly useful in the treatment of coccidiosis.

Tx 8. Tetracyclines

Although this class of drug has reported toxicity, it has widespread use in general practice with few side-effects. It is, however, recommended that this drug is used with great caution, and preferably in conjunction with a probiotic.

   Tetracyclines should only be given orally by dropper and never mixed with the drinking water as there is the risk that in-contact healthy individuals may consume large and toxic amounts of antibiotics as they fulfil their daily water intake.

Dose: 50 mg/kg/day in three divided doses. Alternatively 5 mg/kg can be injected intramuscularly twice a day.

Tx 9. Trimethoprim

Trimabac 20 tablets (Vericore)

These contain 20 mg trimethoprim and 100 mg sulphadiazine sodium.

Dose: These can be crushed to a powder and one-quarter of a tablet given daily to an adult guinea pig. Alternatively the dose can be divided and one-eighth of a tablet given twice daily.

Borgal 7.5% (Hoechst Roussel Vet Ltd.)

This contains 12.5 mg/ml trimethoprim and 62.5 mg/ml sulfadoxine.

Dose: 0.5 ml/kg daily by subcutaneous or intramuscular injection.

PROBIOTICS

These can be given at the same time as the antibiotic to help protect the gut from the damaging effects which occur as the intestinal bacterial flora are destroyed. Probiotics provide a supply of these natural flora.

Tx 10. Enterodex

Enterodex (Vydex Animal Health Ltd.)

Give 1 g (one-quarter of a teaspoonful) mixed with food or a little water once a day.

Tx 11. Live natural yogurt

This contains *Acidophilus* and *Lactobacillus*. A few drops can be given from a teaspoon twice daily.

Tx 12. Avipro

Avipro (VetArk Health)

This is a water soluble probiotic containing *Lactobacillus acidophilus*, *Enterococcus faecium*, *Saccharomyces* and electrolytes. This can be diluted at a dose of 5 g into 200 ml drinking water, or if syringe feeding; if handrearing orphans, a pinch can be added to every feed.

Tx 13. Vetrumex

This is a cattle preparation which contains bacteria necessary for repopulating the rumen. It also acts as an appetite stimulant in guinea pigs as well as cattle and can be given for this purpose even when antibiotics are not being used.

Dose: One-quarter or one-half a teaspoonful mixed with a little water or rosehip syrup daily. It can be administered twice daily if necessary.

FLUID THERAPY

Tx 14. Normal saline 0.9%

In cases of dehydration this fluid can be administered subcutaneously. 10 ml can be given at any one site in the skin overlying the thorax. Up to 20 ml can be given on any one occasion.

Tx 15. Glucose–saline

5% Glucose with 0.9% saline. This is particularly useful in cases of ketosis or anorexia. It can be used post-operatively to provide rehydration and energy. It can be administered subcutaneously, and up to 10 ml can be given at any one site.

Tx 16. Lectade

Lectade (Pfizer Ltd.)

This preparation is used for oral rehydration. As it contains dextrose it is also very useful as a preventative measure for pregnancy toxaemia if it is used to replace the drinking water.

Lectade is available in powder or liquid form. The latter is the more convenient to use and should be used at a dilution of 20 ml liquid Lectade to 250 ml water.

ANTI-FUNGAL AGENTS

Tx 17. Enilconazole

Imaverol (Janssen Animal Health)

This contains 100 mg/ml enilconazole and should be diluted with luke-warm water 1 part Imaverol to 50 parts water and used as a dip three or four times every 3 days.

Tx 18. Griseofulvin

Grisovin powder and grisovin tablets (Schering-Plough Animal Health)

The powder contains 7.5% griseofulvin, and the tablets 125 mg griseofulvin.

Dose: 25 mg/kg daily. This can be achieved by administering one-fifth of a tablet daily, or by incorporating the powder in the feed at a rate of 10 g/kg of dry feed (equivalent to 0.75 mg/kg griseofulvin). This assumes that the average daily intake of dry food is 30 g/kg bodyweight.

If Grisovin is used to treat an individual guinea pig it is best given orally, and in these circumstances one-eighth of a teaspoonful of Grisovin can be mixed with a small amount of an unsaturated fatty acid supplement (e.g. 0.5 ml Norderm, Norden Laboratories) and given daily.

Comment: Griseofulvin should not be administered to the pregnant animal as it is teratogenic.

Tx 19. Tolnaftate 1%

Tinaderm-M cream (Schering-Plough)

This is a human anti-fungal preparation which also contains nystatin; it can be applied to fungal lesions twice a day until they resolve.

Other topical preparations, e.g. Panolog cream (Tx 25), contain nystatin as one of their components.

ANTI-DIARRHOEAL PREPARATIONS

Tx 20. Kaolin

This substance is available in several preparations, either on its own or in combination with other therapeutic agents.

Tx 21. KLN

This is an infant anti-diarrhoeal preparation, containing light kaolin, fruit pectin, oil of peppermint and sodium citrate.

Dose: 3–4 drops three times daily.

Tx 22. Kaolin–morphine

This combination is useful for painful colics.

Dose: 0.2 ml given three times daily.

TOPICAL PREPARATIONS

Tx 23. Dermisol

Dermisol (Pfizer Ltd.)

This cream contains propylene glycol, malic acid, benzoic acid and salicylic acid. It promotes healing by removing dead and necrotic tissue from affected areas and also has anti-bacterial properties.

Dose: Dermisol can be applied to affected areas two or three times daily until the condition resolves.

The same constituents also make up a multi-cleanse solution which is useful to remove necrotic tissue and promote healing.

Tx 24. Kamillosan

This is a herbal preparation which is particularly useful in the treatment of sore nipples. It has the added advantage of being safe to use even when the young are suckling. A little can be applied to the affected nipples two or three times daily.

Tx 25. Panolog cream

Panolog cream (Novartis Animal Health UK Ltd.)

This contains triamcinolone acetonide (potent steroid), neomycin and thiostrepton (antibiotics), and nystatin (anti-fungal).

It is a useful preparation for dermatitis and mixed infections which are accompanied by severe inflammation and pruritus. It can be applied up to three times a day. It is particularly useful for treating scabs around the mouth.

Tx 26. Vetsovate

Vetsovate (Schering-Plough Animal Health)

This contains 0.1% betamethasone (steroid) and 0.5% neomycin (antibiotic). It is useful for bacterial infections accompanied by inflammation and pruritus. It can be applied to the affected area two or three times a day.

EYE PREPARATIONS

Antibiotic only

These should be used when there is corneal damage. There are various preparations available.

Tx 27. Cephalonium

Cepravin eye ointment (Schering-Plough Animal Health)

Apply once or twice a day.

Tx 28. Chlortetracycline

Aureomycin ophthalmic ointment (Fort Dodge Animal Health)

This contains 1% chlortetracycline hydrochloride and can be applied up to three times a day.

Antibiotic and steroid

These can be used for conjunctivitis where there is no accompanying corneal damage.

Tx 29. Neomycin and hydrocortisone

Neobiotic HC (Pharmacia and Upjohn Ltd.)

This preparation is formulated as readily flowing drops and is therefore easier to administer than creams to some patients. Apply three to six times daily.

ECTOPARASITIC PREPARATIONS

Tx 30 Seleen

Seleen (Sanfoni Animal Health Ltd.)

This is a green suspension containing 1% selenium sulphide. It has both anti-parasitic and anti-fungal properties, and is useful for the simultaneous treatment of dermatomycoses and external parasites. It is also beneficial if extensive seborrhoea is present.

The whole guinea pig should be wetted, and the shampoo applied and worked to a lather. The shampoo should be left on the coat for at least 5 minutes before rinsing. Treatment can be repeated weekly as necessary, or more frequently if the condition is severe.

Tx 31. Ivermectin

Ivermectin injection (Merial Animal Health)

This product contains 1% w/v ivermectin. It is not licensed for guinea pigs and must be used with care. It is, however, a very effective ectoparasitic agent.

The dose is 200 µg/kg and this can be repeated at 10–14 day intervals as necessary. The dose of the cattle injection is 0.02 ml/kg, so it is best diluted 1 : 10 with water for injection to produce a more convenient dose of 0.2 ml which should be administered subcutaneously.

Alternatively, the drug can be given orally in its undiluted form. One drop from a 2 ml syringe is equivalent to 200 µg and up to 2 drops can be administered to an adult guinea pig with no adverse side-effects.

Trials at the Cambridge Cavy Trust have shown that larger doses of ivermectin can be given without any adverse side-effects. Their recommendations are as follows:

- Age 3 weeks to 3 months: 0.1 ml by subcutaneous injection. Oral dosing not recommended
- Age 3 months onward: 0.2 ml by subcutaneous injection. One drop given orally

Ivermectin has been administered safely to pregnant sows.

ENDOPARASITIC PREPARATIONS

Tx 32. Metronidazole

Flagyl suspension (May and Baker Pharmaceuticals)

This contains 40 mg/ml of active metronidazole. It is used to treat diseases caused by anaerobic organisms and is also effective against *Trichomonas* spp.

The dose is 20 mg/kg daily given in the drinking water for 7–10 days. The correct dose will be given if 1 ml of Flagyl suspension is mixed with 150 ml of drinking water.

The active ingredient of Torgyl (Tx 4) is also metronidazole.

Tx 33. Piperazine

Antepar elixir (Wellcome Medical Division)

This will effectively control nematodes at a piperazine dose of 3 mg/ml of water. Antepar contains 150 mg piperazine per ml; 1 ml of Antepar should be diluted to 50 ml with water, and this solution used to replace the drinking water for a day.

Tx 34. Praziquantel

Droncit (Bayer)

This will effectively control cestodes at a dose of 5–10 mg/kg orally or 5 mg/kg given by subcutaneous injection.

Tx 35. Sulphadimidine

Intradine (Norbrook Laboratories Ltd.)

This contains 33.3% w/v sulphadimidine and is a useful preparation for the treatment of coccidiosis. It is given in the drinking water at a concentration of 0.2% for 5 days. This concentration will be achieved by diluting 1 ml of Intradine to 150 ml with water.

MISCELLANEOUS TREATMENTS

Tx 36. Atropine

Atropine sulphate injection (Vericore)

This contains 600 µg/ml.

Dose: For premedication: 60 µg/kg. For organophosphate poisoning: 100 µg/kg. Both these should be given by subcutaneous injection.

Tx 37. Betamethasone

Betsolan (Schering-Plough Animal Health)

This is a steroid preparation with powerful anti-inflammatory properties. It can be used in the treatment of pregnancy toxaemia, and the glucogenic effect it produces will last for several days.

Dose: 0.1–0.2 ml given by subcutaneous or intramuscular injection.

Comment: Steroids should not be administered in early pregnancy as they have been shown to cause foetal abnormalities. There is also a risk that they may cause abortion in late pregnancy, but their beneficial effect in the treatment of ketosis outweighs this slight risk.

Tx 38. Dexamethasone

Dexafort (Intervet UK Ltd.)

This combination of long- and short-acting steroid produces a rapid and long-lasting glucogenic effect, and is very important in the treatment of pregnancy toxaemia (ketosis). This drug also has a long-lasting anti-inflammatory and anti-pruritic effect and can be useful in the treatment of skin conditions which are accompanied by intense pruritus.

Dose: In cases of ketosis 0.1 ml should be administered intramuscularly. For the treatment of any other conditions the same dose can be administered subcutaneously.

Comment: The same comments apply for dexamethasone as for betamethasone (see Tx 37).

Tx 39. Doxapram hydrochloride

Dopram-V (Fort Dodge Animal Health)

This contains 20 mg/ml of doxapram hydrochloride, and it is a useful respiratory stimulant.

Dose: 10–15 mg/kg by subcutaneous or intramuscular injection.

Tx 40. Hexetidine

Hexocil (Parke Davis)

This contains 0.5% hexetidine as a shampoo. It has anti-bacterial and anti-fungal properties, and is especially useful in cases with severe seborrhoea of fungal origin. When used to treat fungal conditions it should be in contact with the skin for up to 2 hours before rinsing.

Tx 41. Oxytocin

Oxytocin-S (Intervet UK Ltd.)

One ml contains 10 oxytocin units. The dose to stimulate uterine contractions and milk let-down is 1–2 units, i.e. 0.1–0.2 ml injected intramuscularly.

Tx 42. Primidone

Mysoline suspension (Schering-Plough Animal Health)

This contains 50 mg/ml primidone.

Dose: 0.5 ml/kg twice daily orally.

Tx 43. Tarlite

Tarlite is a tar-based shampoo which is of particular use in cases of seborrhoea, whatever the primary cause of the condition.

It should be used as a shampoo, and applied to the coat once it is wet and then left on the coat for 2–3 minutes before it is rinsed off well. Treatments can be repeated weekly for as often as is necessary.

Tx 44. Diazepam

Valium (Roche)

A dose of 1–2 mg/kg can be given intramuscularly to produce a calming effect in cases with intense pruritus or to those mothers which are initially very apprehensive of their young.

VITAMIN PREPARATIONS

Tx 45. Multivitamin drops

Abidec drops (Parke Davis)

These drops contain vitamins A, C, D and vitamin B complex. Up to 2 drops (0.1 ml) can be given daily to an adult; the dose for a young animal is 1 drop per day.

Abidec drops are useful to ensure adequate vitamins for convalescent animals. Two drops contain 10 mg of vitamin C which is adequate for maintenance of a guinea pig weighing 1 kg. If further vitamin C is required it must be included as an extra supplement.

Tx 46. Colloidal calcium/vitamin D

Collo-Cal D (C-Vet)

This contains 0.75% w/v colloidal calcium oleate and 70 iu/ml of vitamin D.

Dose: 0.5 ml/kg orally once a day.

Tx 47. Vitamin C

Redoxon (Roche)

Soluble vitamin C tablets containing 1000 mg. One tablet should be dissolved in 8 litres of water to produce the required concentration. Tablets are therefore best divided and added to smaller amounts of water. In instances of increased requirements (e.g. pregnancy) one 1000 mg tablet can be dissolved in 5 litres of water.

If vitamin C is being given to treat a clinical case of deficiency it should be given at a rate of 100 mg/kg. In this instance one-tenth of a tablet can be dissolved in a very small amount of water and administered orally.

The diluted solution should be given in glass dishes or drinking bottles with stainless steel nozzles. The breakdown of ascorbic acid is accelerated if it comes into contact with any other metals. Alternatively the required amount (80 ml of the diluted solution) can be mixed in a bran mash.

Tx 48. Vitamin B$_{12}$

This is a very useful vitamin for use in convalescence, and in cases of debilitation or inappetance.

Dose: 0.25 ml of vitamin B$_{12}$ 250 µg given by subcutaneous or intramuscular injection. Treatment can be repeated weekly if necessary.

CLEANSING SOLUTIONS

Tx 49. Hydrogen peroxide

This is very useful for flushing out wounds and abscesses. It should be used at a concentration of 3%.

Tx 50. Povidone–iodine

Povidine antiseptic solution (BK Veterinary Products)

This contains 1% active iodine and it has anti-microbial action against bacteria, fungi, yeasts and some viruses.

It can be used in its concentrated form on wounds, mange, fungal and bacterial infections. It can also be used dilute as a bathing solution, mixed 1 : 5 with water.

Tx 51. Savlon

Savlon Veterinary Concentrate (Schering-Plough Animal Health)

This has antiseptic and anti-bacterial properties and is a useful skin cleaning agent. It should be diluted 1 : 30 in water for use.

Tx 52. Salt solution

The most readily available all purpose bathing solution is a teaspoon of common salt dissolved in a pint of warm water.

12 ALTERNATIVE THERAPIES

Homeopathic and herbal remedies have a definite place in guinea pig medicine, either as an adjunct to conventional medicine, or as an alternative therapy. Veterinary surgeons should use their clinical judgement as to the best combination of therapy (conventional/alternative) for each individual case. Many wild plants have medicinal properties, and where applicable their use may have been mentioned elsewhere in the text, but all homeopathic, herbal and plant remedies are detailed together in this chapter for ease of reference.

HOMEOPATHY

Homeopathic treatment is based on the principle of 'like cures like'. The remedies are substances that are serially diluted, and then used to treat the very symptoms that large amounts of the substance would cause. The most readily available remedies are available in potencies of 6c, 12c, and 30c, where c stands for centesimal dilution. The more dilute a substance is the more potent it is considered to be. 30c is more dilute than 6c and therefore more potent. In general, higher potencies are selected for acute conditions whilst lower potencies are used for more chronic conditions. Many practitioners rely solely on lower potencies (6c) for general use.

Homeopathic remedies for oral use are formulated in tablet or liquid form. When they are administered it is important that they are absorbed through the oral mucosa. Liquids can be given in the drinking water or orally via a dropper. Tablets should be crushed between two spoons and the resultant powder sprinkled into the mouth. The tablets should not be handled as they will absorb moisture and lose their effectiveness. Remedies should not be mixed with the food. When it is necessary to give more than one remedy they should be given at least 5 minutes apart. Tinctures can be used topically, but should not be used undiluted on the skin.

The frequency of administration will depend upon the condition that is being treated. Generally, acute conditions require a high frequency of administration (up to one dose an hour for the first six doses) whilst chronic cases are dosed less frequently (one to three doses daily).

COMMON HOMEOPATHIC REMEDIES

Aconite

6c or 30c. A single dose can be given for shock, or the sudden onset of illness.

Alfalfa

30c. Useful for sows with large litters and little milk. A single dose can be given every few hours until lactation is increased.

Arnica

6c, or 30c or cream. Useful for any form of physical trauma. Can be used for bruising, shock, physical trauma and soft tissue damage. It can be given after a difficult parturition, or following any surgical procedure. The cream should not be applied to broken skin. Treatment should be frequent initially.

Arsenicum album

6c. Used for hot dry itchy skin, where there may be seborrhoea and open sores. One dose can be given two or three times daily until the condition begins to resolve.

Belladonna

30c. Used for acute mastitis, characterized by the sudden onset of pain, heat and swelling of one or both teats. One dose should be given every 2 hours until the condition starts to improve.

Bryonia

6c. This can also be used for mastitis, alongside belladonna. It is useful if the gland is very hard and swollen in the acute stage of the disease.

Calendula

6c, tincture, ointment, cream. This promotes healing of damaged tissue in open wounds. The mother tincture can be diluted 1 : 10 with previously boiled water and used as a skin wash.

Caulophyllum

6c or 30c. This can be used in labour. It eases the dilation of the cervix in the first stage of labour, and strengthens the contractions in the second stage. It may also ease labour pains. It can be given before, during and after the birth where necessary.

Euphrasia

Mother tincture. 3 drops can be mixed with 10 ml of previously boiled water and the solution used as an eye wash.

Gelsemium

6c. This is used for animals that are fearful of noises, or are shy and timid in nature.

Graphites

6c. This can be used for cracked skin with a dry crusty discharge such as scabs around the mouth and lips. It is also suitable for fungal infections.

Hepar sulphuris

6c or 30c. This is useful for the treatment of abscesses. The high potency should be used before the pus has accumulated or come to a head, whereas the low potency will aid the discharge of pus. For this it can be given three times daily for 3 days. This treatment can be followed up with silica 6c.

Hypericum

30c. This can be given in the case of injuries involving nerve damage. One tablet can be given three times a day for the first few days following the injury.

Psorinum

30c. This is made from the human scabies mite. It can be given in cases of mange to aid in the management of the pruritis. One tablet can be given daily for 3 days.

Pulsatilla

6c. Can be used in skin conditions of hormonal origin.

Sabina

12c. This can be used for retained placentas associated with haemorrhage, or for haemorrhage after a miscarriage or abortion. One dose can be given every hour for four doses.

Secale

12c. This can be given in cases of retained placentas associated with a brown, foul smelling discharge. One dose can be given three times a day until the condition improves.

Sepia

6c. This is used for fungal skin conditions, and for hormonal alopecia associated with pregnancy.

Silica

6c and 30c. The low potency is useful for infected wounds, particularly if the wounds have contained foreign bodies. It can also be used to promote the healing of abscesses after the use of hepar sulph. One dose can be given daily for 5 days. The 30c can be used for chronic mastitis, if the gland is hard and the milk caseous. One dose can be given three times a day for 3 days.

Sulphur

6c. This is a common remedy for the treatment of skin conditions. It is most effective if used sparingly. It can be used for both dry skin conditions, and wet, moist lesions. It can help control the open lesions associated with the pruritus caused by mange.

Urtica

6c and 30c. This can be used in lactation. The high potency is used to promote lactation in cases of agalactia. Single doses can be given every few hours until lactation commences. The low potency can be used to depress the milk where necessary.

HERBAL REMEDIES

Many plants and herbs have medicinal properties, and these can be given as an alternative or as an adjunct to conventional treatments. The plants and herbs can be collected and fed fresh, or purchased in a dried or powdered form. The leaves, flowers and stalks of a plant can be made into an infusion by being steeped in boiling water. Herbs can also be made into alcoholic tinctures, or herbal creams. Several herbs with similar properties can be combined to produce powders or tinctures, and these can be administered orally, or via the food or drinking water.

MEDICINAL PLANTS

Agrimony (*Agrimonia eupatoria*)

The whole plant may be fed. It is astringent and has tonic properties. It contains iron, vitamins B and K, and essential oils. It is also a diuretic.

Avens (*Geum urbanum*)

The whole plant can be fed. It is astringent and has tonic properties.

Borage (*Borago officinalis*)

This plant has expectorant, tonic and anti-inflammatory properties. It can help reduce the body temperature in febrile individuals. It can stimulate milk production in lactation.

Bramble (*Rubus fruticosus*)

The common blackberry; its leaves are available for feeding all year round. The leaves are one of the best treatments for scours, and if the guinea pig is otherwise bright, a diet of hay and bramble leaves may be all that is needed to resolve the condition.

Chickweed (*Stellaria media*)

The whole plant may be fed. It has anti-rheumatic, astringent and anti-pruritic properties.

Cleavers (*Galium aparine*)

More commonly known as 'goosegrass' this plant is diuretic, anti-inflammatory, tonic and astringent. It can be used in cases of renal or bladder calculi, and for skin complaints.

Clover (*Trifolium* spp.)

The whole plant can be fed. It is a good source of vitamins, minerals and proteins. Its also has tonic properties.

Coltsfoot (*Tussilago farfara*)

The leaves of the plant can be fed. It has expectorant, anti-tussive, demulcent and anti-catarrhal properties, and has a reputation as a curer of coughs and chest complaints. It also reduces irritation and inflammation throughout the gastrointestinal system and prevents diarrhoea. It reduces peristalsis by relaxing the gut lining.

Comfrey (*Symphytum officinale*)

Comfrey is astringent and has expectorant properties. It is a useful adjunct in the treatment of respiratory infections as it can help remove mucus from the respiratory tract.

Cornsilk (*Zea mays*)

This plant is rich in polyunsaturated fatty acids, and is diuretic, demulcent and a tonic. It can be used for urinary tract infections and renal calculi.

Dandelion (*Taraxacum officinale*)

The whole plant can be fed. It has a diuretic action and a stimulating effect on the kidney. The leaves can be fed to help eliminate bladder stones. It is also laxative in action and should generally be fed sparingly.

Echinacea (*Echinacea augustifolia*)

This is currently popular as a supplement used to increase resistance to infection and to support the immune system. It can be given to guinea pigs with systemic illness to help recovery. It is the root of the plant that has medicinal properties.

Fennel (*Foeniculum vulgare*)

Fennel stimulates peristalsis, relaxes the stomach and can help relieve the symptoms of bloat. Fennel can also help stimulate milk production during lactation.

Garlic (*Allium sativum*)

Garlic has antiseptic, hypotensive and antispasmodic properties. It is one of the most effective anti-microbial plants available, as is said to act on bacteria, viruses and alimentary parasites. It may help maintain the normal balance of gastrointestinal flora, by supporting the natural bacteria and acting against pathogenic species. Garlic can be used externally as a wound wash. Garlic also has anti-catarrhal properties and can be used as an adjunct to the treatment of respiratory infections.

Goat's rue (*Galega officinalis*)

This herb has a powerful action on the mammary glands, stimulating their development and increasing their milk supply.

Groundsel (*Senecio vulgaris*)

The whole plant can be fed. It is a tonic and laxative, and is a good source of minerals.

Parsley (*Petroselinum crispum*)

Parsley is diuretic, relieves bloat, and is a good appetite stimulant. It may also increase milk production in lactating sows. It is a reproductive stimulant and if fed before breeding may lead to increased litter size. It should be avoided in the later stages of pregnancy, as it is a womb stimulant.

Plantain (*Plantago* spp.)

There are two types of plantain, the broad-leaved greater plantain and the narrow-leaved ribwort plantain. All parts of the plant may be fed. They have astringent and diuretic action. Plantains have an anti-inflammatory action on the gut lining, and help prevent diarrhoea. They are a useful adjunct to the treatment of scours. Plantains are also said to have an anti-microbial action, and help the body resist, and fight off, infection.

Raspberry (*Rubus idaeus*)

Raspberry leaves are astringent and have tonic properties. They also have an action on uterine muscles, and if fed throughout the last third of gestation are thought to lead to easier births. They may also stimulate milk production during lactation. Raspberry also has anti-inflammatory properties and can help reduce the body temperature in febrile individuals.

Shepherd's purse (*Capsella bursa-pastoris*)

All parts of the plant can be fed, and it can be dried and stored and used during the winter. It is astringent and one of the best plants available to treat scouring. It also has tonic properties, has a stimulating effect on the womb, and can be used to help prevent excessive post-partum bleeding.

Sow thistle (*Sonchus oleraceus*)

The whole plant can be fed; the hollow stems exude a milky sap, and they are an ideal food for lactating sows.

Wild carrot (*Daucus carota*)

The seeds contain volatile oils which are a urinary antiseptic, useful in the treatment of cystitis and urolithiasis. It may help in treatment of arthritis. The roots are a good source of vitamin C and carotene.

Willow (*Salix* spp.)

The leaves can be fed. They have aspirin-like properties and are useful during the recovery from surgery, or other painful conditions.

Yarrow (*Achillea millefolium*)

This plant is astringent, and of value in the treatment of scours. It is also a diuretic, is of value as a urinary antiseptic, and can be given in cases of cystitis. Yarrow also has anti-catarrhal properties and can be used as an adjunct to the treatment of respiratory infections.

13 ZOONOTIC ASPECTS

Guinea pigs are generally kept in close association with humans, as the majority of them are children's pets or kept by the hobbyist for breeding and exhibiting. Although there are several potential zoonotic organisms which may affect guinea pigs they are seldom associated with human disease.

Ringworm

This is the most common zoonosis as the fungal spores are transferred when the guinea pig is handled. The most frequently isolated dermatophyte is *Trichophyton mentagrophytes*, and lesions on the owner are usually found on the hands and arms.

Proven or suspected cases of ringworm should only be handled for the administration of treatment, and gloves should be worn for this procedure. Any spores on in-contact bedding can be destroyed by burning, and the hutch can be cleaned with a 2% formalin solution, or with a dilute solution of enilconazole (Tx 17).

Mange

Mange caused by *Trixacarus caviae* is probably the most frequent skin complaint of guinea pigs. However, human skin disease caused by this mite is very rare, presumably because this mite is a burrowing mite and not immediately accessible for transmission. Extra precautions are not usually necessary during the treatment of affected individuals.

Salmonellosis

This zoonosis has the most public health significance, but thankfully *Sal-*

monella spp. are rare pathogens for guinea pigs. However, when *Salmonella* spp. are isolated, the whole caviary should be depopulated. Healthy animals which are not in-contact can be removed and isolated, but affected animals and those which recover should be destroyed. Recovered animals are likely to become carriers and therefore perpetuate the disease.

All premises, feeding and drinking utensils should be thoroughly disinfected with a 5% formalin solution or other approved disinfectant, and all bedding and hay destroyed by burning.

Yersiniosis (pseudotuberculosis)

This disease is also rarely seen in guinea pigs. However, when diagnosed all affected animals should be destroyed and all premises and utensils well disinfected.

In humans *Yersinia* can cause a rare mesenteric lymphadenitis and enteritis, the signs of which are similar to acute appendicitis.

Allergic responses to guinea pigs

Some owners may develop asthma-like symptoms after being in close association with guinea pigs. The allergen may be their hair or skin debris, but more commonly is the hay and the owner develops a condition akin to 'farmer's lung'. Avoiding the use of mouldy or dusty hay, and the wearing of a facemask whilst in the caviary should minimize the symptoms.

Other allergy symptoms which have been reported in laboratory technicians and other personnel working in close association with guinea pigs are rhinitis and skin rashes.

APPENDIX 1: MISCELLANEOUS PHYSIOLOGICAL DATA

Body temperature (rectal thermometer)	38.3–40°C (100–104°F)
Heart rate	230–320/minute
Respiration rate	90–150/minute
Tidal volume	2–5 ml/kg
Blood volume	6% of body weight
Life expectancy	Up to 8 years, usually 4–5 years
Environmental temperature	20–22°C (optimum performance)
	15–18°C (acceptable average)

Digestive parameters

Food intake	6 g per 100 g body weight of which 2–4 g is dry food. They eat 8% of their body weight as dried food
Water intake	85 ml/day (average adult). Approximately 8 ml/100 g body weight
First eat solid food	2–4 days old

Reproductive parameters

Sexual maturity (female)	4–6 weeks
Sexual maturity (male)	4–6 weeks
Female breeding age	4–5 months, weight 500 g
Male breeding age	3–5 months, weight 550 g
Oestrus cycle	15–17 days
Ovulation	Spontaneous – approximately 10 hours after onset of oestrus
Gestation period	59–72 days (depending upon litter size)
Litter size	1–6 (average 3)
Birthweight	75–100 g

Breeding life of female   4–5 years
Breeding life of male   5 years or longer
Lactation period   3 weeks
Weaning age   3 weeks

Haematology

Blood sampling: Small samples can be collected by overclipping a toe-nail; 0.25 ml can be obtained by venesection of the marginal ear vein.

Blood volume (ml/kg body weight)   75
Haematocrit   37–48
Haemaglobin (g/dl blood)   11–17.2
RBC count (per ml) $4.5–7 \times 10^6$
WBC count (per ml) $3.2–15 \times 10^6$
   Neutrophils   28–44% (average 37%)
   Lymphocytes   39–72% (average 56%)
   Eosinophils   1–5%
   Monocytes   3–12%
   Basophils   0–3%

APPENDIX 2: SUMMARY OF HERBAL AND HOMEOPATHIC REMEDIES AND THEIR USES

The Digestive System

Diarrhoea	Agrimony, avens, bramble and raspberry leaves, plantain, yarrow
Constipation	Cleavers, dandelion, groundsel
Bloat	Fennel, garlic
Hepatic stimulants	Agrimony, celery, cleavers, dandelion, fennel, yarrow

The Respiratory System

Expectorants	Chickweed, coltsfoot, comfrey, mallow, plantain
Anti-catarrhals	Garlic, yarrow

The Reproductive System

Labour	Raspberry, caulophyllum
Miscarriage/retained placenta	Sabina, secale
Post-partum bleeding	Secale, shepherd's purse
Agalactia	Alfalfa, urtica, borage, fennel, sow thistle, parsley, raspberry
Mastitis	Belladonna, bryonia

The Skin

Abscesses	Hepar sulphuris, silica
Pruritus	Arsenicum album, chickweed
Seborrhea	Arsenicum album, sulphur
Mouth scabs	Graphites
Mange	Psorinum
Hormonal	Pulsatilla, sepia
Fungal	Sepia

Non-specific lesions   Sulphur
Wounds–healing   Calendula
infected   Silica

The Urinary System
Diuretics   Agrimony, borage, cleavers, cornsilk,
                              dandelion
Cystitis   Cornsilk, yarrow

Miscellaneous
Shock   Aconite
Trauma   Arnica
Nerve damage   Hypericum
Fear   Gelsemium
Pyrexia   Borage, plantain, raspberry
Immune system stimulants   Echinacea, garlic, plantain

FURTHER READING

Anderson, L. (1987) Guinea pig husbandry and medicine. *Veterinary Clinics of North America* **17**, 1045–59.

Axelrod, J. (1980) *Breeding Guinea pigs*. TFH Publications, USA.

Buckland, M.D., Hall, L. *et al.* (1981) *A Guide to Laboratory Animal Technology*. Heinemann, USA.

Cooper, G. and Schiller, R.L. (1975) *Anatomy of the Guinea Pig*. Harvard Press, USA.

Elward, M. (1980) *Encyclopedia of Guinea Pigs*. TFH Publications, USA.

Flecknell, P. (1983) Restraint, anaesthesia and treatment of children's pets. *In Practice* May, 85–95.

Flecknell, P. (1985) *Guinea Pigs. Manual of Exotic Pets*. BSAVA, 36–44.

Harkness, J. (1994) Guinea pig biology and medicine, North American Veterinary Conference, Orlando, FL.

Harkness, J.E. and Wagner, J.E. (1989) *The Biology and Medicine of Rabbits and Rodents*. Lea and Febiger, Philadelphia.

Hillier, E.V. and Quesenberry, K.E. (1997) *Ferrets, Rabbits and Rodents, Clinical Medicine and Surgery*. W.B. Saunders Company, USA.

Hime, J.M. and O'Donoghue, P.N. (1979) *Handbook of Diseases of Laboratory Animals*. Heinemann.

Hutchinson, P. (1978) *Guinea Pigs, Their Care and Breeding*. K and R Books.

Laber-Laird, K. Swindle, M. and Flecknell, P. (1996) *Rodent and Rabbit Medicine*. Pergamon Press, Oxford.

Lawrence, K. (1987) Facts and data to help the treatment of smaller domestic pets. *The Henston Veterinary Vade Mecum*. 337–40.

The Merck Veterinary Manual (1979) Merck, New Jersey.

Sebesteny, A. (1976) Diseases of guinea pigs. *Veterinary Record* **98**, 418–23.

Turner, J. (1981) *Exhibition and Pet Cavies*. Spur Publications.

Universities Federation for Animal Welfare (1999) *The UFAW Handbook on the Care and Management of Laboratory Animals*. Blackwell Science, Oxford.

Wagner, J.E. and Manning, P.J. (1976) *Biology of the Guinea Pig*. Academic Press, New York.

Williams, C.S.F. (1979) Guinea pigs and rabbits. *Veterinary Clinics of North America* **9**(3), 487–97.

Yeatts, J.W.G. (1994) Rabbit fur mite. *Veterinary Record* **134**, 359–60.

INDEX